Praise for

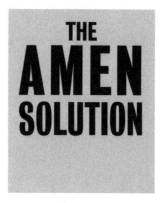

THE
AMEN
SOLUTION

"A masterful analysis of the factors that influence weight gain and permanent, sustainable weight loss, written in easy-to-understand language, leaving the reader with only one thought: 'I can do this!'"

—Dr. David Ajibade, cofounder and
president of Building Strength, LLC

"I've witnessed the positive results of *The Amen Solution* both personally and with my patients. This is a book you will want to get for yourself, your friends, family, and the health care professionals in your life! Help change the world and join the brain health revolution."

—Earl R. Henslin, Psy.D., author of *This Is Your Brain on Joy*

"A great book, filled with good, solid, simple advice for eating healthy and losing weight, with many original strategies for interrupting negative behaviors and enhancing motivation—key elements for achieving success."

—Andrew Newberg, M.D., and Mark Robert Waldman,
authors of *How God Changes Your Brain*

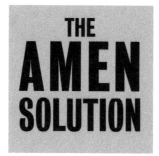

THE AMEN SOLUTION

The Brain Healthy Way to
Lose Weight and Keep It Off

DANIEL G. AMEN, M.D.

The Secret to Being Thinner,
Smarter, Happier

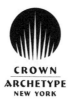

CROWN
ARCHETYPE
NEW YORK

MEDICAL DISCLAIMER

The information presented in this book is the result of years of practice experience and clinical research by the author. The information in this book, by necessity, is of a general nature and not a substitute for an evaluation or treatment by a competent medical specialist. If you believe you are in need of medical interventions, please see a medical practitioner as soon as possible. The stories in this book are true. The names and circumstances of the stories have been changed to protect the anonymity of patients.

Published in the United States by Crown Archetype, an imprint of the Crown Publishing Group, a division of Random House, Inc., New York.

www.crownpublishing.com

Crown Archetype with colophon is a trademark of Random House, Inc.

Library of Congress Cataloging-in-Publication Data is available upon request.

ISBN 978-0-307-46360-9
eISBN 978-0-307-46362-3

Printed in the United States of America

Book design by Helene Berinsky

Jacket design by Jennifer O'Connor

Jacket photograph by Blake Little

10 9 8 7 6 5 4 3 2 1

First Edition

To Matt, I am rooting for you

CONTENTS

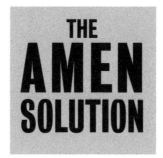

THE
AMEN
SOLUTION

INTRODUCTION

In my book *Change Your Brain, Change Your Body,* I wrote about how you can use your brain to improve the health of your heart, skin, energy, focus, memory, sexual function, and weight. In it, I revealed that based on our brain imaging work at the Amen Clinics with tens of thousands of patients from eighty different countries over the last twenty years, we have discovered two of the major secrets why most diets don't work. And contrary to what you might think, they have nothing to do with your lack of desire to lose weight or your willpower. In fact, for some people the harder they try to lose weight, the worse it gets.

The first secret is that most weight problems occur between your ears. So stapling your stomach may, in fact, be working on the wrong organ. Not to mention that ten years after gastric banding surgery, the success rate is a disappointing 31 percent. It is your brain that pushes you away from the table telling you that you've had enough, and it is your brain that gives you permission to have that second bowl of ice cream, making you look and feel like a blob. *If you want a better body, the first place to always start is by having a better brain.*

The second secret, based on our brain imaging work, is that there is not just *one* brain pattern associated with being overweight; there are at least five different patterns. Giving everyone the same diet plan will make some people better and a lot of people worse. Knowing about your own specific brain will make losing weight and keeping it off a whole lot easier.

The response to these revelations has been amazing, and the book vaulted onto the *New York Times* bestseller list and stayed there for months. I knew people would respond to the message that their brain and weight are intricately connected and that if you boost your brain you can have a better body. What I wasn't prepared for, though, was the deluge of desperate requests from readers asking for more specific help on how to use their brains to lose their bellies.

Ever since *Change Your Brain, Change Your Body* hit cyberspace and store shelves, people have been calling and e-mailing our clinics; posting comments on my blog; and talking to me at book signings, speaking engagements, and other events. What the overwhelming majority of them were begging for was a simple step-by-step brain-based program for weight loss.

The Amen Solution: The Brain Healthy Way to Lose Weight and Keep It Off is that program.

I like to call it weight loss for thoughtful people. This is definitely not weight loss for dummies. As you know, there are a lot of dumb ways to try to lose weight. You may have even tried some of them. You know the kinds of methods I am talking about—the cookie diet, mustard diet, eat anything you want for an hour a day diet, cabbage soup diet, part-time diet (one day on, one day off), grapefruit diet, baby food diet, liquid diet, juice detox diet, coconut oil diet, ice cube diet, ice cream diet, grape diet, eat only one kind of food per meal diet, caveman diet, red wine diet, pizza diet, one-day diet, three-day diet, seven-day diet, peanut butter diet, and even the tapeworm diet (yes, some people are actually willing to swallow a tapeworm to try to lose weight). These types of gimmicky diets promise fast results—"Lose 10 pounds in seven days!"—but are more likely to set you up for failure in the long run.

My favorite story about dumb ways to lose weight came from one of my public television appearances. When I got to one of the stations for a live on-air appearance, a colleague I will call Jim, with whom I had worked before, looked thinner. I asked Jim what he was doing. He told me he was on the hCG diet. Human chorionic gonadotropin is a pregnancy hormone that, in conjunction with a 500-calorie-a-day diet *(yikes!)*, has been reported to help people with rapid weight loss. The placebo-controlled studies with hCG have been less than impressive. Nonetheless, my friend did very well on the diet, losing 20 pounds. It is a diet you can only do for twenty-six days at a time because people seem to become immune to its effects. On the last day of the diet, as a way to celebrate his weight loss, Jim told me he called his favorite deep-dish pizza restaurant in Chicago and ordered two large deep-dish pizzas that he planned to gorge on over the weekend.

When he told me this story, I looked at him like he was the dumbest person on the planet. "You're kidding me, right?" I asked as I looked into his eyes.

"No, why?" he replied defensively.

"You are acting like an alcoholic who just got out of rehab, and as a way to celebrate, you are going to get drunk!" Not exactly a sign of intelligent life.

When I saw him several months later, he had put back on all the weight he had lost.

The Amen Solution for Anxiety and Depression Also Helps Your Weight

The seeds for this book came from two projects at the Amen Clinics. First, a few years ago I wrote a twelve-week home study course for conquering anxiety and depression, using principles I had been teaching for years at the Amen Clinics. There is good scientific evidence that many people can improve their mood and decrease their level of anxiety by implementing specific strategies at home.

When I was on the follow-up calls with our ninety participants, the majority of people told me they felt less anxious and less depressed, which I had expected, but what I didn't expect was that some people told me that they had also lost 10, 20, and even 30 pounds in the twelve weeks and found that their memory and focus were better as well. In listening to those calls I had an "aha" moment and realized that with a better brain you also get a better body and a better mind.

Science backs up this discovery. Research presented at the annual meeting of the Society of Ingestive Behavior in 2009 found that depressed patients who followed a six-month behavioral weight-loss program not only lost weight but also reported a significant drop in their symptoms of depression. Lose weight, get happier.

Amen Clinic NFL Brain Imaging / Rehabilitation Program Helps Players Lose Weight and Get Smarter

The second project that's helped seed this book is my work in performing the world's largest brain imaging / brain rehabilitation study on active and retired professional football players. We have evaluated and treated more than one hundred players. For many years, the NFL has said that it didn't know if playing professional football caused long-term brain damage. After a number of players came to see me with dementia, depression, and obesity, I decided to study their brains and answer once and for all the question "Does playing football damage the brain?" The answer, which did not surprise anyone except perhaps some in the NFL, was *of course playing professional football causes long-term brain damage.* You cannot get hit by guys like Minnesota Viking Ron Yary (6'5" and 255 pounds) thirty to fifty times a game and not expect to have some trouble.

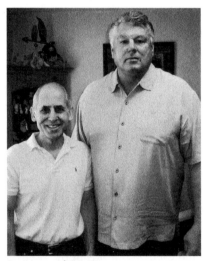

Dr. Amen and Ron Yary

But the exciting news is that when we put our players on our brain healthy program, many of them not only lost weight (one of our players lost over 100 pounds), they also got smarter and happier at the same time. Plus, their cognitive scores improved, sometimes by 200, 300, or even 400 percent.

Here is an example: Big Ed White, age sixty-two, a four-time Pro Bowl offensive guard for the Minnesota Vikings and later for the San Diego Chargers, played seventeen seasons in the National Football League. When I first met Ed he weighed 365 pounds and scored very poorly on his cogni-

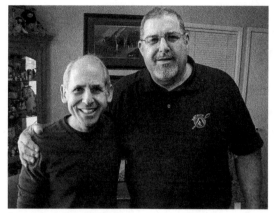

Dr. Amen and Big Ed White

tive testing profile. All of our players take a test called the Microcog, which measures intellectual functioning in nine different areas, including overall general cognitive functioning, information processing speed, attention, reasoning, and memory. He scored very poorly. After six months on our brain healthy / weight-loss program, he had lost 40 pounds, and his test scores increased dramatically (see below).

ED WHITE'S MICROCOG RESULTS			
	Before	**After**	**% Change**
General cognitive functioning	21	39	90%+
Information processing	25	58	> 100%+
Reasoning	3	13	> 400%+
Memory	14	66	> 470%+

The numbers are Ed's percentile rankings, comparing him with other people his age and education level. For example, a ranking of 21 percent means 79 percent of people his age and education scored better than Ed.

Our research with the NFL players also demonstrated what other researchers had found: *As your weight goes up, your brainpower goes down.* Below is a graph of what happens to our players' reasoning scores as their weight—measured by body mass index (BMI)—goes up. It should make anyone be concerned about their weight.

Research has clearly shown that obesity increases your risk for Alzheimer's disease and other forms of dementia. Plus, Cyrus Raji's group at the University of Pittsburgh found that the brains of overweight people—people with a BMI between 25 and 30—had 4 percent less volume than the brains of people with lower BMIs, and their brains looked eight years older than healthy people's. People who were obese—people with a BMI over 30 (Ed White's BMI when he first came to see us was 45) had 8 percent less brain volume, and their brains looked sixteen years older than healthy people's.

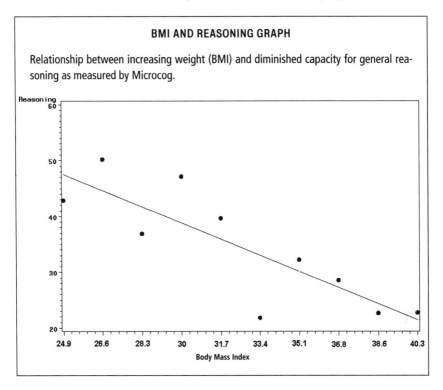

BMI AND REASONING GRAPH

Relationship between increasing weight (BMI) and diminished capacity for general reasoning as measured by Microcog.

THE PROMISE AND THE PROGRAM

In this book I will give you the basic steps to boost your brain to become thinner, smarter, and happier at the same time. I will give you a ten-week program to get started. This is the same program we use at the Amen Clinics, and the same program we use with our NFL players. Take note that we started our weight-loss pilot program on December 1, and everybody told us we were crazy to conduct a weight-loss study over the holidays when most people tend to gain weight. But we wanted to make sure our program could stand up to real-life challenges, like holiday feasts and treats. It did. Our group actually lost on average 2.8 pounds during the week of Christmas! On average, our participants lose 10 pounds in ten weeks. (Note that individual results may vary.) Many of our participants have lost much, much more.

- **Eileen,** fifty-five, lost 15 pounds in ten weeks, but after three ten-week cycles she lost 39 pounds, and she reported that she felt happier and smarter. "It made a big change in my whole life."
- **Dan** lost 39 pounds in ten weeks, 50 pounds after his second ten-week cycle, and a total of 69 pounds after his third ten-week program and reports he is happier and in much more control of his whole life. He told us, "This diet was so much easier than the ones in the past because the cravings were actually gone."
- **John** lost 35 pounds in ten weeks and says he is a happier, more fun person to be around.
- **Amy** lost four pant sizes and said it was much easier than she suspected it would be. She tells her friends that healthy food is medicine.
- **Betty** lost 16 pounds and says when she goes out to eat with her husband they get one plate and split it, and when she walks out of the restaurant she no longer feels stuffed and stupid.
- **Rhona** was already at a healthy weight to start and took the course just to support a friend, but she ended up losing 5½ pounds after ten weeks and then another 4 pounds after the following ten-week program. She said, "This has changed my life. I thought when I took the course I might learn something and lose a pound or two, but I never thought it would change my life. And personally for me, when I am shopping, I now think, does this feed my brain? That was something I had never thought of before."

Throughout the pages of this book, you will learn much more about these and many other participants in our weight-loss program, including several of our NFL players. In "The Amen Solution All-Stars" profiles, these real-life people will share their personal journeys to a slimmer shape, greater happiness, and improved brain function. I hope their stories will inspire and motivate you.

You will also find "Get Smart to Get Thinner" boxes with thoughtful tips, strategies, insights, and success stories from the everyday people who have been successfully losing weight with this program. These quotes come from our weight-loss program participants as well as people who have posted comments on my blog or posted online reviews of my book *Change Your Brain, Change Your Body.* I have changed their names to protect their privacy and have edited some of the quotes for space and clarity.

Why ten weeks to start? You need at least seventy days to change bad habits and to start solidifying good ones. However, this is not a ten-week program. This is a program to get control of your brain and your body for *the rest of your life.* Ten weeks is just a start. If you act like hCG, Chicago deep-dish pizza Jim in the story relayed earlier, you will never get it right. Here is a summary of the program.

STEP 1: THE AMEN SOLUTION OVERVIEW—DO THESE TEN THINGS FIRST!

Immediately, I will give you the basic steps of the program, so you can get started immediately, including what important numbers you need to know and start improving right away, plus how to keep a daily journal to help your brain develop new neuronal networks to help direct your behavior in a positive way.

STEP 2: KNOW YOUR MOTIVATION TO GET HEALTHY

To lose weight and keep it off, you must be able to maintain a high level of motivation. In this step I will focus and enhance your desire to be healthier, happier, and smarter.

STEP 3: EAT RIGHT TO THINK RIGHT AND KEEP TRACK OF WHAT YOU EAT

Food is medicine and can help you be trim, vibrant, happy, and focused, or it can make you plump, sluggish, sad, and stupid. In this step I will give you the Amen Clinics Seven Rules for Brain Healthy Eating. Journaling is a critical part of the program to be successful, so you keep a record of what you put into your body to avoid calorie amnesia.

STEP 4: KNOW YOUR BRAIN TYPE

By now, you have learned our basic steps to lose weight and be happier and smarter, but not everyone is the same. In this section I will explore the five different types of overeaters, the interventions for each type, and what to do if you have more than one type.

STEP 5: TAKE BRAIN HEALTHY SUPPLEMENTS

Nutritional supplementation can enhance weight control, mood, focus, and memory. Here I will explore a rational scientific approach to using supplements, including ones I think most people should take and ones that may better fit your individual situation.

STEP 6: LEARN NINE SECRETS TO CONQUERING YOUR CRAVINGS

Cravings are usually what sabotages most people's success in dieting. In this step I will give you nine secrets to getting control of your cravings to increase the chances this program will be successful.

STEP 7: REV YOUR METABOLISM

Both physical and mental exercises are essential to weight loss and a brain healthy life. In this step I will explore the right kinds of physical exercise that rev your metabolism and how new learning also boosts brain metabolism.

STEP 8: KILL THE ANTS

Negative thinking patterns make you fat, mentally sluggish, and unhappy. Here I will give you an in-depth look at correcting the automatic negative thoughts, or ANTs, that drive depression and overeating.

STEP 9: PRACTICE DIRECTED FOCUS

Both hypnosis and meditation are powerful tools to enhance brain and body function. I will teach you simple exercises to enhance your brain and your body.

STEP 10: BUST YOUR BARRIERS

There are many barriers that derail success. Here I will give you simple tools to prevent relapse, stop other people from making you fat, and information on what to do after you reach your ideal weight.

In addition, there is a questionnaire to help you know your type, and many, many tools to help you stay on track for success, including two hundred ways to leave your blubber behind, calorie counts, a grocery shopping list, brain healthy recipes, and flash cards of brain healthy reminders you can cut out and keep with you at all times. On our website, you'll find even more interactive tools to help you reach your goals.

Boosting your brain to get slimmer, smarter, and happier is a big promise. Follow me for at least ten weeks and let me prove it to you. What do you have to lose? More of your belly while you get a better brain!

THE AMEN SOLUTION

DO THESE TEN THINGS FIRST!

Whenever I have read a book about nutrition and weight loss, it seemed that I had to hunt for the essence of the program throughout the book. That really irked me. I would think to myself, "Hey, give me a summary! Make this easy for me. I want to get started today." So here is the Amen Solution, in as simple language as possible to help you get started today. The Amen Solution is a brain-centered weight-loss program designed to help you get thinner, smarter, and happier at the same time. The rest of the book explains everything you need to know to make this happen in more detail.

1. Know your important numbers.
2. Know your motivation to get healthy.
3. Eat right to think right and keep track of what you eat.
4. Know your brain type.
5. Take brain healthy supplements.
6. Learn nine secrets to conquering your cravings.
7. Rev your metabolism.
8. Kill the ANTs.
9. Practice directed focus.
10. Bust your barriers.

1. Know Your Important Numbers

When it comes to the health of your brain and body, there are some numbers that are critical to know. When some of these numbers are out of whack, it can prevent you from losing weight, keep you in the dumps, and reduce brain function. Optimizing these numbers can be one of the keys to helping you achieve your weight-loss goals, feel happier, and boost your brainpower. The Amen Solution will help you optimize these numbers throughout the first ten weeks on the program and beyond. Here are some important numbers you need to know to maintain a healthy brain and body.

As you begin your journey, it is a good idea to take stock of your numbers. Then at the end of the ten weeks, check these numbers again to see how much progress you have made. You can track your numbers in our *Change Your Brain, Change Your Body Daily Journal* or online on our website.

GET SMART TO GET THINNER

"It works! Optimize your brain . . . and willpower, priorities, and focus are yours! I've lost 35 pounds and I'm looking at losing another 25, and I *know* I can do it!"

—Allie

BODY MASS INDEX

This number tells you the health of your weight based on your height. A normal BMI score is between 18.5 and 24.9; between 25 and 29.9 is overweight; between 30 and 39.9 is obese; and over 40 is morbidly obese. As I mentioned in the introduction, Dr. Cyrus Raji and colleagues from the University of Pittsburgh found that *people who were overweight, who had a BMI between 25 and 30, had 4 percent less brain tissue and their brains looked eight years older than healthy-weight people! People who were obese, who had a BMI over 30, had 8 percent less brain tissue, and their brains looked sixteen years older than healthy-weight people!*

To be healthy, happy and smart, you have to get your BMI under control. For a free BMI calculator, go to www.amenclinic.com.

One of the reasons why I want my patients to know their BMI is that it stops them from lying to themselves about their weight. I was sitting at dinner recently with a friend who seemed totally indifferent about his weight, even though he was injecting himself with insulin for his diabetes at the table. As we were talking, I calculated his BMI for him. Trust me, I can be a very irritating friend if I think you are not taking care of yourself. His BMI was just over 30, in the obese range. That really got his attention, and since then he has lost 20 pounds and is more committed to getting healthy. The truth will set you free. Know your BMI.

WAIST-TO-HEIGHT RATIO

Another way to measure the health of your weight is called your waist-to-height ratio (WHtR). Some researchers believe this number is even more accurate than your BMI. BMI does not take into account an individual's frame, gender, or the amount of muscle mass versus fat mass. For example, two people can have the same BMI, even if one is much more muscular and carrying far less abdominal fat than the other; this is because BMI does not account for differences in fat distribution.

The WHtR is calculated by dividing waist size by height and takes gender into account. As an example, a male with a 32-inch waist who is 5'10" (70 inches) would divide 32 by 70, to get a WHtR of 45.7 percent. The WHtR is thought to give a more accurate assessment of health since the most dangerous place to carry weight is in the abdomen. Fat in the abdomen, which is associated with a larger waist, is metabolically active and produces various hormones that can cause harmful effects, such as diabetes, elevated blood pressure, and altered lipid (blood fat) levels.

Many athletes, both male and female, who often have a higher percentage of muscle and a lower percentage of body fat, have relatively high BMIs, but their WHtRs are within a healthy range. This also holds true for women who have a "pear" rather than an "apple" shape.

The following chart helps you determine if your WHtR falls in a healthy range (these ratios are percentages):

WOMEN
- Ratio less than 35: Abnormally slim to underweight
- Ratio 35 to 41.9: Extremely slim
- Ratio 42 to 48.9: Healthy
- Ratio 49 to 53.9: Overweight
- Ratio 54 to 57.9: Seriously overweight
- Ratio over 58: Highly obese

MEN
- Ratio less than 35: Abnormally slim to underweight
- Ratio 35 to 42.9: Extremely slim
- Ratio 43 to 52.9: Healthy
- Ratio 53 to 57.9: Overweight
- Ratio 58 to 62.9: Seriously overweight
- Ratio over 63: Highly Obese

GET SMART TO GET THINNER

"I started out in a 2X then went down to a 1X to an XL to an L. Now I'm wearing the same pants size I was in high school."

—Lisa

KNOW YOUR DAILY CALORIC NEEDS TO MAINTAIN CURRENT BODY WEIGHT

I think of calories like money. Wise caloric spending is a critical component to getting healthy. Don't let anyone tell you that calories don't count. They absolutely do. The people who say calories don't matter are just fooling themselves. You need to know how many calories you need to eat a day to maintain your current weight. The average fifty-year-old woman needs about 1,800 calories, and the average fifty-year-old man needs about 2,200 calories a day. This number can go up or down based on exercise level and height. You can find a free personalized "caloric need" calculator at www.amenclinics.com.

DESIRED WEIGHT

Set a realistic goal for your desired weight and match your behavior to reach it. If you wish to lose a pound a week, you typically need to eat 500 calories a day *less* than you burn. I am not a fan of rapid weight loss. It does not teach you how to live for the long term. One of my patients went on the hCG diet I told you about in the introduction and lost 40 pounds in three twenty-six day cycles, but it was at a pretty high cost. Within the next six months, she put all the weight back on plus 10 more pounds. Slow and steady teaches you new habits. At the Amen Clinics our average weight loss in our groups is 10 pounds in ten weeks, but individual results may vary. That helps people be more consistent for the long term.

KNOW THE DAILY CALORIES YOU CONSUME (STOMP OUT CALORIE AMNESIA!)

For the next ten weeks keep a food log and count every calorie that goes into your body. This is just like keeping a budget. If you keep this log, together with the other parts of the program, it will be a major step forward in getting control of your brain and body for the rest of your life. If you don't know the calories of something, don't eat it. Why are you going to let someone else sabotage your health? *Ignorance is not bliss. It increases your chances for an early death.*

You need to learn to weigh and measure food and really look at the food labels for portion size. What the cereal companies think is a portion size may not be anywhere near what your eyes think. When you actually do this, I can promise you it will be a rude awakening. I know it was for me. Upon keeping track of his calories, one of our NFL players wrote, "I had no idea of the self-abuse I was doing to my body!"

KNOW THE NUMBER OF FRUITS AND VEGETABLES A DAY YOU EAT— COUNT THEM

Eat more vegetables than fruits and try to get that number to between five and ten servings to enhance your brain and lower your risk for cancer.

KNOW THE NUMBER OF HOURS YOU SLEEP AT NIGHT

Don't fool yourself into thinking you only need a few hours of sleep. I used to think that I was "special" because I could get by on four or five hours of sleep at night, until I actually read the research. Then I realized I was just dumb. Getting fewer than seven hours of sleep at night is associated with lower overall blood flow to the brain, more cravings, and more fat on your body. No wonder I had trouble losing the extra 20 pounds. Even worse, having chronic insomnia triples your risk of death from all causes. Strive to get seven or, even better, eight hours of sleep every night. Teenagers need to get at least nine hours a night.

GET SCREENING LABORATORY TESTS AND YOUR BLOOD PRESSURE TESTED TO OPTIMIZE YOUR BRAIN AND BODY

Here are tests I order at the Amen Clinics for our weight-loss groups. Ask your health care provider to order these as part of a healthy brain/body program.

- **Complete blood count** This will check the health of your blood. People with low blood count can feel anxious and tired, and they may overeat as a way to medicate themselves. People with alcohol problems may have large red blood cells.
- **General metabolic panel** This will check the health of your liver, kidneys, fasting blood sugar, and cholesterol.

- **Vitamin D level** Low levels of vitamin D have been associated with obesity, depression, cognitive impairment, heart disease, reduced immunity, cancer, psychosis, and all causes of mortality. Have your physician check your 25-hydroxy vitamin D level, and if it is low get more sunshine and/or take a vitamin D_3 supplement. I have to take 10,000 IUs (international units) of Vitamin D_3 a day to keep my levels near high normal.

  > Low: < 30
  > Optimal: 50–90
  > High: > 100

- **Thyroid** An overactive thyroid can mimic symptoms of anxiety that make you want to eat as a way to calm down. Having low thyroid levels decreases overall brain activity, which can impair your thinking, judgment, and self-control and make it very hard for you to lose weight. Have your doctor check your free T3 and TSH (thyroid-stimulating hormone) levels to check for hypothyroidism or hyperthyroidism and treat as necessary to normalize.

- **C-reactive protein** This is a measure of inflammation that your doctor can check with a simple blood test. Elevated inflammation is associated with a number of diseases and conditions and should prompt you to eliminate bad brain habits and get thin. Fats cells produce chemicals called cytokines that increase inflammation in your body.

- **HgA1C** This test shows your average blood sugar levels over the past two to three months and is used to diagnose diabetes and prediabetes. Normal results for a nondiabetic person are in the range of 4 to 5.6 percent. Prediabetes is indicated by levels in the 5.7 to 6.4 percent range. Numbers higher than that may indicate diabetes.

- **DHEA (dehydroepiandrosterone) and free and total serum testosterone level** Low levels of the hormones DHEA and testosterone, for men or women, have been associated with low energy, cardiovascular disease, obesity, low libido, depression, and Alzheimer's disease.

- **Blood pressure** Have your doctor check your blood pressure at your yearly physical or more often if it is high. High blood pressure is associated with lower overall brain function, which means more bad decisions.

KNOW HOW MANY OF THE TWELVE MOST IMPORTANT MODIFIABLE HEALTH RISK FACTORS YOU HAVE, AND THEN WORK TO DECREASE THEM

Here is a list from researchers at the Harvard School of Public Health. Circle the ones that apply to you.

- Smoking
- High blood pressure
- BMI indicating overweight or obese
- Physical inactivity
- High fasting blood glucose
- High LDL cholesterol
- Alcohol abuse
- Low omega-3 fatty acids
- High dietary saturated fat intake
- Low polyunsaturated fat intake
- High dietary salt
- Low intake of fruits and vegetables

2. Know Your Motivation to Get Healthy

In chapter 2 we will spend time working specifically on motivation. For now, know that in order for you to consistently make the right decisions, you must have a burning desire to be healthy. Why do you care?

For me, I have an amazing wife, four wonderful children, and a new grandson, Elias. My grandfather was one of the most important people in my whole life. I was named after him and he was my best friend growing up. I know how important grandparents can be. The day Elias was born I thought about my grandfather all day long. I *want* to be healthy to be able to love Elias like my grandfather loved me. When I really think about what's important to me, no amount of cheeseburgers, sodas, or double-fudge chocolate chip brownies is worth the price of damaging my health and stealing the time I have with my family.

You have to focus on your motivation, or food will control you. Brain imaging studies have shown that many foods that are filled with fat, sugar, and salt actually work on the morphine or heroin centers of our brain and can be totally addictive. An animal study from a team of French scientists found that sugar was actually *more* addictive than cocaine. Many of my overweight patients act just like addicts and spend their days either thinking about food, trying *not* to think about food, or eating. Many food companies are highly skilled in giving you that momentary burst of pleasure, but like with any drug, it is an illusion and if you are not careful, you will get hooked. Bet you can't eat just one!

Many people are going bankrupt because they are living in the moment without any thought toward the future. They aren't using their prefrontal cortex, the area of the brain involved in planning, judgment, and follow-through, to think about the consequences of their actions. *The Power of Now* can kill you early. No offense to Eckhart Tolle, whom I admire and respect very much, but you need to be thinking about how your thoughts and behaviors today impact your brain and body half an hour, a day, a year, ten years, and thirty years from now.

Throughout the program, we will work on what motivates you. Is it health, or is it fear? Some people, me included, require fear. I finally lost the extra 20 pounds because I kept reading studies like the one I mentioned from the University of Pittsburgh. Given that your brain controls everything you do, including how much love you have in your life and how much money you make, you do not want a smaller brain!

GET SMART TO GET THINNER

"After just three weeks, I'm already seeing noticeable improvements. I'm losing weight, sleeping better, and my memory is better."

—Leslie

Remember the graph from the introduction, which showed that *as your weight goes up your reasoning goes down*?

The fat on your body is not just a storage place for excess calories. It promotes inflammation, which can lead to heart disease, diabetes, and Alzheimer's disease. Plus, fat stores toxic materials, which can directly damage your brain. But again, the exciting news is that if you work to get healthy, you can reverse the brain damage. But the sooner the better!

So, you have to ask yourself, "What is my specific motivation to get healthy?" Write it down and put it where you can see it every day. Be positive: I want to live long, have great energy, look great, be smart. If your motivation is like mine and it involves the people you love, put up their pictures where you can see them every day. My screensaver is a photo of me with my grandson Elias.

Focus on the reasons why you must be healthy every day, or the doughnuts

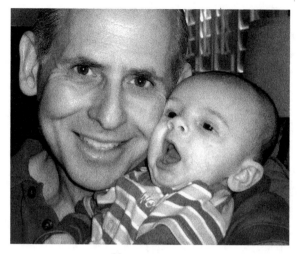

My screensaver

will always win. And doughnuts don't make you sexy! Research suggests that getting a sugar burst can lower your testosterone levels, for men or for women, by up to 25 percent, which decreases your interest in sex. Oh, great! This means that sharing the cheesecake at the restaurant may mean that no one will get dessert when they get home.

3. Eat Right to Think Right and Keep Track of What You Eat

Food is medicine and can help you be trim, vibrant, happy, and focused, or it can make you plump, sluggish, sad, and stupid. It can also help keep you healthy or increase your risk for disease. Did you know that diet accounts for 30 to 35 percent of all environmentally caused cancers? According to William Li, M.D., head of the Angiogenesis Foundation, obesity and cancer are both promoted by something called angiogenesis. Angiogenesis is a natural process in which the body regulates the growth of blood vessels. When this process gets out of control and too many blood vessels grow, myriad diseases can result, including cancer, obesity, and Alzheimer's disease.

Stopping the growth of blood vessels could be useful in the treatment of cancer or obesity, according to Li. A host of antiangiogenic drugs are already on the market, but Li and researchers at the Angiogenesis Foundation have also identified numerous foods that are natural angiogenesis inhibitors. Consuming these foods could play an important role in fighting obesity as well as cancer. Many of the brain healthy foods I write about in this book are also antiangiogenic. Some of them include:

- Apples
- Blackberries
- Blueberries
- Cherries
- Dark chocolate
- Garlic
- Grapefruit
- Green tea
- Lemons
- Nutmeg
- Olive oil
- Oranges
- Raspberries
- Red grapes
- Soybeans
- Strawberries
- Tomatoes
- Tuna
- Turmeric

Overall, you want great value for the calories you consume. In chapter 3 I will go into detail about a brain healthy diet. For now, here are the Amen Clinics Seven Rules for Brain Healthy Eating.

RULE 1. THINK HIGH-QUALITY CALORIES IN VERSUS HIGH-QUALITY ENERGY OUT.

Don't let anyone tell you that calories don't count. They absolutely do. But it is not as simple as calories in versus calories out. I want you to think about eating mostly "high-quality calories." One cinnamon roll can cost you 720 calories and will drain your brain, whereas a 400-calorie salad made of spinach, salmon, blueberries, apples, walnuts, and red bell peppers will supercharge your energy and make you smarter.

"High-quality energy out" means you need to rev up your metabolism in a healthy way. Exercise, new learning, and green tea help. Diet pills, sugary caffeinated energy drinks, excessive coffee (green tea has half the caffeine as coffee), caffeinated sodas, and smoking are low-quality energy boosters.

| GET SMART TO GET THINNER |

"I thought I knew all there was to know about dieting and eating right, but I was wrong. I lost 3 pounds in one week after making some minor changes that were recommended in the first few steps of your program. I feel better than ever."

—Jeri

RULE 2. DRINK PLENTY OF WATER AND NOT TOO MANY OF YOUR CALORIES.

Your brain is 80 percent water. Anything that dehydrates it, such as too much caffeine or too much alcohol, decreases your thinking and impairs your judgment. Make sure you get plenty of water every day. On a trip to New York City recently I saw a poster that read, ARE YOU POURING ON THE POUNDS? DON'T DRINK YOURSELF FAT. I thought it was brilliant. A recent study found that on average Americans drink 450 calories a day, twice as many as we did thirty years ago. Just adding the extra 225 calories a day will put 23 pounds of fat a year on your body, and most people tend to not count the calories they drink.

RULE 3. EAT HIGH-QUALITY LEAN PROTEIN EARLIER IN THE DAY.

It helps balance your blood sugar, boosts concentration, and provides the necessary building blocks for brain health. Great sources of protein include fish, skinless turkey or chicken, beans, raw nuts, low-fat or nonfat dairy, and high-protein vegetables, such as broccoli and spinach. Did you know that spinach is nearly 50 percent protein? I use it instead of lettuce on my sandwiches for a huge nutrition boost.

RULE 4. EAT LOW-GLYCEMIC, HIGH-FIBER CARBOHYDRATES.

This means eating carbohydrates that do not spike your blood sugar and are also high in fiber, such as those found in whole grains, vegetables, and fruits, such as blueberries and apples. Carbohydrates are *not* the enemy. They are essential to your life. Bad carbohydrates are the enemy. These are carbohydrates that have been robbed of any nutritional value, such as simple sugars and refined carbohydrates. If you want to live without cravings, eliminate these completely from your diet. I like the old saying "The whiter the bread, the faster you are dead."

GET SMART TO GET THINNER

"You have to become an expert in reading nutrition labels!"

—John

Sugar is *not* your friend. Sugar increases inflammation in your body, increases erratic brain-cell firing, and has been recently implicated in aggression. In a new study, children who were given sugar every day had a significantly higher risk for violence later in life. I don't agree with the people who say "Everything in moderation." Consuming cocaine or arsenic in moderation is *not* a good idea. The less sugar in your life, the better your life will be.

RULE 5. FOCUS YOUR DIET ON HEALTHY FATS.

Eliminate bad fats, such as all trans fats and most animal fat. Did you know that fat stores toxic materials? So when you eat animal fat, you are also eating anything toxic the animal ate. Yuck. Did you know that certain fats that are found in pizza, ice cream, and cheeseburgers fool the brain into ignoring the signals that you should be full? No wonder I used to always eat two bowls of ice cream and eight slices of pizza!

Focus your diet on healthy fats, especially those that contain omega-3 fatty acids, found in foods like salmon, avocados, walnuts, and green leafy vegetables. High cholesterol levels are not good for your brain. A new study reports that people who had high cholesterol levels in their forties had a higher risk of getting Alzheimer's disease in their sixties and seventies. But don't let your cholesterol levels go too low either. Did you know that low cholesterol levels have been associated with both homicide and suicide? If I am at a party and someone is bragging to me about their low cholesterol levels, I am always very nice to that person.

RULE 6. EAT FROM THE RAINBOW.

This means putting natural foods in your diet of many different colors, such as blueberries, pomegranates, yellow squash, and red bell peppers. This will boost the antioxidant levels in your body and help keep your brain young. Of course, this does not mean Skittles or jelly beans.

RULE 7. COOK WITH BRAIN HEALTHY HERBS AND SPICES TO BOOST YOUR BRAINPOWER.

Here is a little food for thought, literally.

- Turmeric, found in curry, contains a chemical that has been shown to decrease the plaques in the brain thought to be responsible for Alzheimer's disease.
- In four studies a saffron extract was found to be as effective as antidepressant medication in treating people with major depression.
- There is very good scientific evidence that sage helps to boost memory.
- Cinnamon has been shown to help attention. It has also been found to help regulate blood sugar levels, which improves brain function and decision making. Research also shows that cinnamon extract can inhibit the aggregation of tau proteins in the brain, which is associated with Alzheimer's disease. Plus, cinnamon is a natural aphrodisiac for men, not that most men need much help. My wife makes an amazing sweet potato soup with slivered almonds, cranberries, cinnamon, and sage. It makes me smarter and more affectionate at the same time.

Journaling is a critical part of our program. Keeping a food journal helps you avoid calorie amnesia. Writing down everything that goes into your body for ten weeks makes you conscious, aware, and more likely to do the right things. It is easier than ever to do this by using our available journal or an online calorie-counting program. I think journaling what you eat is like keeping a checkbook. It holds you accountable. If you don't know how much money you are spending, you are much more likely to become bankrupt. If you eat or drink more calories than you burn, your body will become fat and nutritionally bankrupt.

4. Know Your Brain Type

When I first started to do our brain imaging work at the Amen Clinics in 1991 I was looking for the *one* pattern that was associated with depression, attention deficit disorder (ADD), or bipolar disorder. But as I soon discovered there was clearly not one brain pattern associated with any of these illnesses. They all had multiple types. Of course, I then realized there will never be just one pattern for depression, because not all depressed people are the same. Some are withdrawn, others are angry, and still others are anxious or obsessive. The scans helped me understand the type of depression, or ADD, or bipolar disorder a person had so that I could better target their treatment. This one idea led to a dramatic breakthrough in my own personal effectiveness with patients and it opened up a new world of understanding and hope for the tens of thousands of people who have come to the Amen Clinics and the millions of people who have read my books.

As we looked at the brains of our overweight patients, we discovered that again there was not one brain pattern associated with being overweight; there were at least *five* patterns. We saw patterns associated with brains that tended to be compulsive, some were impulsive, others were sad, and still others anxious, in various combinations. This is exactly the reason why most diets don't work. They take a one-size-fits-all approach, which, based on our brain imaging work, makes absolutely no sense at all.

Take the test questionnaire in appendix A of the book to see whether or not you fit into a type or types. If you do, read chapter 4 to learn more about your type and what you can do about it. Here is a brief summary of each type. Most people will never need a brain scan to know their type.

Brain Type 1 Is "the Compulsive Overeater"

People who are this type tend to get stuck on the thought of food and feel compulsively driven to eat. They often say that they have no control over food and tend to be nighttime eaters because they worry and have trouble sleeping. Compulsive overeaters generally have too much activity in the front part of their brains, usually due to low levels of a chemical called serotonin, so they overfocus and can get stuck on the same thought, such as the ice cream in the freezer that is calling their name.

Caffeine and diet pills usually make people with this type anxious, because their brains do not need more stimulation, and they often feel as though they need a glass of wine at night, or two or three, to calm their worries. Compulsive overeaters do best when we find natural ways to increase serotonin. Serotonin is calming to the brain. Physical exercise boosts serotonin as does using certain supplements, such as 5-HTP, saffron, inositol, L-tryptophan, or St. John's Wort. There is good scientific evidence that 5-HTP (5-hydroxytryptophan) can be helpful for weight loss, and in my experience, I have found it to be especially helpful for this type.

Brain Type 2 Is "the Impulsive Overeater"

People with this type have poor impulse control, get distracted easily, and just reach for food without thinking. Their brain scans show low activity in the front part of the brain in an area called the prefrontal cortex. Think of the prefrontal cortex like the brain's brake. It stops us from saying stupid things or making bad decisions. It is the little voice in your head that helps you decide between the banana and the banana split.

GET SMART TO GET THINNER

"I have taken your test, and it has been revealed that I am probably an impulsive overeater. Tears came to my eyes because my prayers have been answered just to know that the reason I am having difficulty reaching my goal weight is because I have been using the wrong approach."

—Lana

Impulsive overeating is common among people who have attention deficit disorder (ADD), which has been associated with low dopamine levels in the brain. People with ADD struggle with a short attention span, distractibility, disorganization, and impulsivity. Research suggests that having untreated ADD nearly doubles the risk for being overweight. And, without proper treatment, it is nearly impossible for these people to be consistent with any nutrition plan. Overweight smokers and heavy coffee drinkers also tend to fit this type.

We help impulsive overeaters by boosting dopamine levels in the brain and strengthening the prefrontal cortex. Higher-protein, lower-carbohydrate diets tend to help, as does exercise and certain stimulating medications or supplements, such as green tea or L-tyrosine. Any supplement or medicine that calms the brain, such as 5-HTP, typically makes this type *worse* because it can lower both your worries and your impulse control.

GET SMART TO GET THINNER

"I found out that the supplements I had been taking for years might not be the best for my brain type. So I switched and am doing much better."

—Karen

Brain Type 3 Is a Combination of Types 1 and 2 and Is Called "the Impulsive-Compulsive Overeater"

On the surface, it seems almost contradictory. How can you be both impulsive and compulsive at the same time? Think of compulsive gamblers. These are people who are compulsively driven to gamble and yet have very little control over their impulses. It is the same with these overeaters. Our scans tend to show too much activity in the brain's gear shifter, so people overthink and get stuck on negative thoughts, but they also have too little activity in the prefrontal cortex so they have trouble supervising their own behavior. People with this type benefit from treatments that increase both serotonin and dopamine, such as exercise with a combination of supplements like 5-HTP and green tea.

Brain Type 4 Is "the Sad or Emotional Overeater"

People with this type overeat to medicate their feelings of sadness and to calm the emotional storms in their brains. They often struggle with depression, low energy, low self-esteem, and pain symptoms, and they tend to gain weight in winter. Their brain scans tend to show too much activity in the limbic or emotional part of the brain. For this type, exercise, fish oil, optimizing their vitamin D level, and certain supplements, such as SAMe (S-adenosylmethionine) can be very helpful to balance the brain, improve your mood, help with energy, and decrease pain.

Brain Type 5 Is "the Anxious Overeater"

People with this type medicate their feelings of anxiety or nervousness with food. They often complain of waiting for something bad to happen and frequently suffer from headaches and stomach problems. Their brain scans often show too much activity in an area called the basal ganglia. This part of the brain is involved in setting a person's anxiety level. When there is too much activity here, because of low levels of a chemical called GABA (gamma-aminobutyric acid), people often have anxiety and a lot of physical tension. The best treatment for this type is to soothe the brain with meditation and hypnosis, plus using a combination of vitamin B_6, magnesium, and GABA.

It is common to have more than one brain type. If that is true for you, work on the most bothersome brain type first and then go on to the others. I will address this issue later in the book.

5. Take Brain Healthy Supplements

According to recent studies, more than half of Americans do not eat at least five servings of fruits and vegetables a day, the minimum required to get the nutrition you need. I recommend that all of my patients take a good multiple vitamin/mineral supplement every day plus omega-3 fatty acids. When weight is an issue, I recommend supplements that can help with cravings (more on this in a bit) and ones that may benefit your specific type of brain. The thoughtful use of supplements is an essential part of a healthy brain plan.

For example, according to researchers at the Harvard School of Public Health mentioned above, having low levels of omega-3 fatty acids is one of the leading preventable causes of death and has been associated with heart disease, strokes, depression, suicidal behavior, ADD, dementia, and obesity. Taking fish oil, a good source of omega-3s, has been found to be good for your heart, your skin, your eyes, your joints, your hair, and your brain. In a recent study, taking omega-3s has also been found to decrease your appetite and your cravings. My recommendation for most adults is to take between 1–2 g (grams) of high-quality fish oil a day. When we put our retired football players on our fish oil supplements, many of them were able to decrease or completely eliminate their pain medications.

Another critical supplement is vitamin D. Low levels of vitamin D have been associated with depression, Alzheimer's disease, multiple sclerosis, heart disease, diabetes, cancer, and obesity. When you don't have enough vitamin D, you feel hungry all the time, no matter how much you eat. Typically, we get a vitamin D boost from the sun, but because we are wearing more sunscreen and spending more time inside in front of our computers, our levels are falling and our health is at greater risk. And it is an easy fix. Have your doctor order a test called 25-hydroxy vitamin D, and take vitamin D_3 if your levels are low. Of course, supplements will never work by themselves if you eat too much or do not exercise. To be smart, you have to do the whole program, including knowing your brain type. There is much more on the thoughtful use of supplements later in the book.

6. Learn Nine Secrets to Conquering Your Cravings

As already mentioned, fish oil and vitamin D can help decrease your cravings. Here are some of the nine ways brain science can help.

KEEP YOUR BLOOD SUGAR BALANCED

Low blood sugar levels are associated with lower overall brain activity. Low brain activity means more cravings and more bad decisions. The supplements alpha-lipoic acid and chromium have very good scientific evidence that they help balance blood sugar levels and can help with cravings. In addition:

- Eat a healthy breakfast. People who maintain weight loss eat a nutritious breakfast.
- Have smaller meals throughout the day.
- Stay away from simple sugars and refined carbohydrates, such as candy, sodas, cookies, crackers, white rice, and white bread.

GET SMART TO GET THINNER

"You have changed my life forever! Just a year ago, I weighed in excess of 550 pounds. Within six months, I am down to under 400 pounds and am still going strong."

—Richard

KILL THE SUGAR OR IT WILL KILL YOU

High-sugar, high-fat foods work on the addiction centers of your brain. When I finally got this idea through my own thick skull it made a *huge* difference for me. I *love* living without cravings. But for years I fought the idea of giving up sweets, like candy or Rocky Road ice cream. I thought it was simply about calories in versus calories out. If I stayed within a certain calorie range, I would be fine. The problem was that eating the sugar activated my cravings and made it very hard to stay away from things that were bad for me.

Sweets are mood foods for me. My grandfather was a candy maker and my best memories growing up were standing at the stove next to him making fudge or pralines. But my grandfather was also overweight and had two heart attacks that took him away from me way too early. I know that kicking the sugar habit isn't easy for many people. It is like kicking a drug, and it certainly wasn't easy for me. But I found that when I substituted brain healthy fruit like blueberries, bananas, and apples, the cravings completely went away. Have you ever known someone to eat too many bananas? For most people, it takes about two weeks of completely avoiding sugar for your cravings to go away.

GET SMART TO GET THINNER

"I have begun making permanent changes in my life and am already noticing a dramatic difference! My moods have improved and I've already noticed an increase in my energy level."

—Caroline

DECREASE THE ARTIFICIAL SWEETENERS IN YOUR DIET

We think of these sweeteners as free, because they have *no* calories, but because they are up to six hundred times sweeter than sugar they may activate the appetite centers of the brain, making you crave even more food. Diet sodas are *not* the answer. The one natural no-calorie sweetener I like is called stevia, but it should still be used sparingly.

DAILY STRESS-MANAGEMENT PROGRAM

Anything stressful can trigger certain hormones that activate your cravings, making you believe that you need that cinnamon roll. Meditation and hypnosis are wonderful stress-management practices that can help boost your brain and decrease your stress and your weight. More on these shortly.

OUTSMART THOSE SNEAKY FOOD TRIGGERS THAT TRY TO SABOTAGE YOU NEARLY EVERYWHERE YOU GO

If you go to the mall, the airport, or the ball game, you will see store after store and vendor after vendor selling things that will make you fat and unhappy. For example, whenever I went to the movies, I used to immediately think about getting a big tub of popcorn with lots of butter along with red licorice until I actually thought about the saturated fat, salt, sugar, and artificial dye that would be flooding my brain. To control your cravings, you have to control your triggers. Know your vulnerable times and plan ahead. I take a snack with me when I go to the movies so that I am not tempted by the popcorn and candy.

HIDDEN FOOD ALLERGIES CAN ALSO TRIGGER CRAVINGS AND MAKE YOU FAT

For example, did you know that wheat gluten and milk allergies can decrease blood flow to the brain and decrease your judgment? In chapter 6, I will show you how to use a simple elimination diet to know what foods you may or may not be sensitive to.

7. Rev Your Metabolism

Physical and mental exercise are two critical components of our plan and will be explored in detail later. For now, walk at least four times a week for forty-five minutes and try to learn something new every day.

GET SMART TO GET THINNER

"When you eat healthy brain food, get rid of the ANTs, and meditate, then exercise and hunger control become easy."

—Stephen

---

8. Kill the ANTs

Being overweight or being unhappy are "thinking disorders," not just eating or mood disorders. ANTs stands for "automatic negative thoughts," the thoughts that come into your mind automatically and ruin your day. I think of these negative thoughts like ANTs that infest your psyche and ruin your body. You need to develop an internal ANTeater to patrol the streets of your mind. Most people don't know that their thoughts can lie. For most of us, they typically lie a lot. And it is your uninvestigated thoughts that will kill you early.

Many of our retired NFL players are obese when they first enter our study. One of my favorite players, Big Ed White from the Minnesota Vikings, weighed 365 pounds when I first met him. When I asked him about his weight, he told me that he had no control over his eating. That was his automatic response: "I have no control." "Is that true?" I asked. "You really have *no* control over your eating?"

He paused and said, "No. That really isn't true . . . I do have some control."

"But just by thinking that you have no control," I said, "you have just given yourself permission to eat anything you want at any time you want."

Another obese player told me that he just didn't like any of the foods that were healthy for him. "Is it really true," I countered, "that you don't like any of them?" I then showed him a list of our fifty best brain healthy foods, and in fact, he liked about 60 percent of them.

Another player told me that everyone in his family was overweight. It was just his genetics. "Is that true?" I pressed. "Are you saying that this really doesn't have anything to do with how much you eat? My genes say I am supposed to be fat too. Your genes are not your destiny." He then looked at me and said, "That's a pretty lame excuse, isn't it?"

It is the little lies that you tell yourself, like "I have no control" or "It is my genetics," that make you fat and steal your health and happiness. One of the most important steps in winning the battle of the bulge is to get control of your mind. In chapter 8 we will go into ANT-killing techniques in great detail. For now, whenever you feel anxious, sad, obsessive, or out of control, write down the automatic thoughts that are going through your mind. The act of writing them down helps to get them out of your head. Then ask yourself if the thoughts make sense, if they are really true. For example, if you hear yourself thinking, "I have no control," write that down. Then ask yourself, "Is it true? If someone held a gun to my head, would I still really have to eat that piece of French apple pie?"

You do not have to believe every stupid thought that goes through your brain. This method of challenging your thoughts to help your weight is backed by strong scientific evidence. Researchers from Sweden found that the people who were trained to talk back to their negative thoughts lost 17 pounds in ten weeks and continued to lose weight over eighteen months, proving this technique works over the long term.

GET SMART TO GET THINNER

"By following the steps in this program, I am consistently losing weight, and I feel so much better!"

—Jason

---

9. Practice Directed Focus

There is very good scientific evidence that when you add hypnosis or meditation to a healthy weight-loss program, you can improve the outcome. For those of you with a busy mind, like mine, both hypnosis and meditation can calm your thoughts and increase self-control. In one study that we performed at the Amen Clinics sponsored by the Alzheimer's Research & Prevention Foundation, we found that a very simple twelve-minute meditation boosted blood flow to the front part of the brain, which enhances judgment and decision making.

Likewise, I have found few things as immediately helpful as hypnosis to change behavior and help understand the emotional reasons for overeating. If you have experienced emotional trauma, then hypnosis, meditation, and psychotherapy can be very helpful. A set of hypnosis CDs and meditation exercises can be found at www.amenclinics.com.

10. Bust Your Barriers

To be successful at boosting weight loss, happiness, and IQ, it is critical to overcome the barriers that derail success. In chapter 10 I will show you how to prevent relapse and not allow others to make you fat and stupid. I will also give you a plan on what do to after you get to your ideal weight. For now do not let yourself get:

- Too hungry (keep a balanced blood sugar)
- Too angry (losing control of your emotions will often trigger overeating)
- Too lonely (humans do better when they have the company and support of others)
- Too tired (good sleep is essential to getting control of your appetite, cravings, and brain health)

GET SMART TO GET THINNER

"I have been struggling with weight loss for the past eight years. I have tried everything from diet pills to hypnosis. With this program though, I went from 251 pounds to 228 pounds in eight weeks."

—Petra

Now that you have the general outline of the program, meet Dan, one of the Amen Solution All-Stars, to show you how he puts it all together.

The Amen Solution All-Stars: Dan

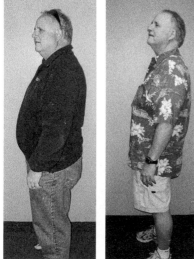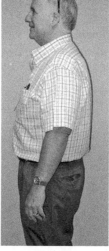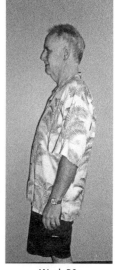

| Before, 274 pounds | Week 10, lost 39 pounds | Week 20, lost 50 pounds | Week 30, lost 69 pounds |

Dan, fifty-five, used to think about food *all day long*! That's very common among Type 1 Compulsive Overeaters like him. Before the program, he really had no clue how many calories a day he ate and suffered from intense cravings for things like bread, potatoes, New York steak, and chili. "Just driving down the road, McDonald's would call out to me," he admitted.

He tried diet after diet, but nothing ever worked, and he couldn't curb his cravings. Now he understands why. "Some of the diet programs were really good rah-rah fun, but they sold so many products with ingredients like enriched flour, sugar, and artificial sweeteners. Through this program, I've learned that eating those things actually *increases* cravings," he said. Dan was so frustrated by his inability to lose weight he was actually considering getting LAP-BAND surgery. Then he heard about our weight-loss group.

When he joined the Amen Solution program, he weighed 274 pounds and his short-term goal was just to "keep from putting on more weight during the holidays." He did far more than that! He lost 50 pounds in just two ten-week cycles and a total of 69 pounds after three ten-week cycles, bringing him down to 205 pounds.

He accomplished this, in part, by knowing his important numbers, including his BMI, which was 38 when he started. As I write this book, his BMI is down to 28. For Dan, discovering his brain type and understanding underlying problems were other big steps in solving his weight struggle. With the tools in this program, he said he has "learned to combat the compulsion, anxiety, and mood swings that have caused my overeating." And for the first time in his life, he said, "The refrigerator has stopped calling me."

Dan really got the message of "high-quality calories in versus high-quality energy out." He counts his calories in the *Daily Journal* and weighs his food. He focuses on healthy foods that add great value to his body. He has cut out simple sugars and artificial sweeteners and uses the natural sweetener stevia instead. He stopped drinking caffeine and alcohol and is now exercising on a regular basis. He takes a multiple vitamin, fish oil, vitamin D, and our Craving Control formula, which he says "takes the edge off dieting." He also loves our Focus & Energy Optimizer supplement as a replacement for caffeine.

He also started eating breakfast every day. "I used to get up and have coffee, but I wouldn't eat anything. It wouldn't faze me until I was starving to death and then would pound down a huge lunch," he said. "Now I make sure to eat something every morning—a banana, an apple, a little oatmeal, just something. I end up eating less throughout the day."

Dan has also discovered how to modify his old favorite fat-filled recipes to make them more brain healthy. "I love chili, but now I make it with organic tomatoes, pinto beans, and portobello mushrooms instead of ground beef. I actually like it better than the way I used to make it," he said.

Weight loss isn't the only thing Dan gained from his new brain healthy habits. He said he now feels healthier and more alert, and his memory has improved. He said he has even gotten his temper under control. "I've noticed that the road rage I used to feel while driving has gone way down."

2

KNOW YOUR MOTIVATION
TO GET HEALTHY

DRIVE YOUR DESIRE TO CHANGE

"I don't have time."

"I don't have the energy to exercise."

"I don't like any of the foods that are healthy for me."

"I feel bad when I eat right. I just want the ice cream, pizza, and cheeseburgers too much."

"I'll start tomorrow, or Monday, or next week, or next month . . . if I ever really get sick."

"I can't keep a food journal."

"I have no control over what I eat."

"My family won't support me."

Sound familiar? Most of us are experts at coming up with excuses why we can't change our behavior. Change is hard. At first, any change is challenging, which is why most people do not do it. Our brains resist change. When we do the "same old things" our brains can basically cruise on autopilot without much effort. Our brains get comfortable with our daily habits and routines, even if they are unhealthy for us. For us to change our habits, the brain has to be rewired and develop a whole new system, and it fights that process. That's why even though you know that you should stop gorging on the French fries, you don't do it.

But change is not as hard as you think. For me, I found that when I did this whole program, the change actually came easily and gradually. I lost 20 pounds over about twenty weeks. I like the idea of slow weight loss (even for the impatient among us), because if you do it slowly, then it is becoming part of a lifestyle change that you can maintain. The quick-weight-loss programs cause you to deprive yourself and suffer for a few weeks or months, and then it is back to the bad habits.

You have to follow all ten steps to make this work. Weight will not come off by wishful thinking. You will not be happier by willing yourself so, and you certainly will not be smarter by just taking a supplement. Getting healthy requires good planning and focused energy.

To make lasting progress, you must know what's motivating you to be healthy. Why do you care? For you to break free from the habits that have been keeping you fat, unhappy, and not functioning at your intellectual potential, you must know your motivation. Is it to:

- Prevent disease?
- Live longer?
- Be a better role model for your children?
- Have greater self-esteem?
- Be more confident in bed?
- Look younger?
- Look better in jeans?
- Be able to participate in sports and other activities you used to enjoy?
- Have a better relationship with your spouse?
- Reverse diabetes, heart disease, or other health risks?
- Decrease your risk for Alzheimer's disease?
- Stop beating yourself up about your weight?
- Have the confidence to apply for the job you really want?
- Impact your emotional and spiritual health?

What is your specific motivation to change? Write it down and put it where you can see it every day. Be positive or use negative reasons, whatever works for you.

Positive reasons might include:

"I want to live longer."
"I want to have more energy."
"I want to look great."
"I want to feel better."
"I want to have better relationships."
"I want to be happier and smarter for the long run."

On the negative side, reasons might include:

"I want to avoid getting diabetes and having my legs amputated like my dad did."
"I don't want the kids pointing at me ever again, saying I'm fat."
"I never want to feel like I don't fit in."
"I want to avoid being embarrassed taking my clothes off in front of my husband."

If your motivation involves the loved ones in your life, put their pictures up where you can see them. Use the "My Motivation" page here or create a personal page on our website to create your own daily motivation reminder.

MY MOTIVATION

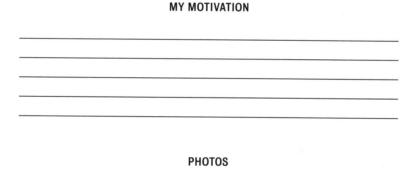

PHOTOS

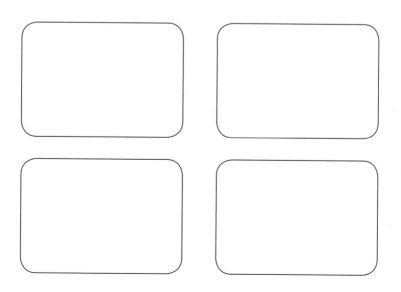

The First Step to Change Is Pain

*"The day I was diagnosed with diabetes, it scared me so much I stopped
eating sugar."*

*"When I found out I was pregnant, I was terrified my daughter would grow
up to be miserable and fat like me."*

"After I had a heart attack, my doctor told me I had to change my diet."

*"My mother died at age fifty-four from a stroke, and I didn't want to be
next."*

*"When the airline made me buy two seats for my size, I couldn't take the
humiliation."*

"The depression overwhelms me. I have to change."

"My memory is awful and I am afraid it is going to get worse."

For many overweight people, it takes something drastic, like a heart attack
or a diagnosis of diabetes, to inspire change. Typically, it is only when your
unhealthy habits cause enough pain in your life that you finally make the
decision to change.

You know how powerful pain can be. On a day when you feel fine, there
is no way you would spend eight dollars for a bottle of one hundred aspirin,
but if you have a killer headache, you would gladly fork over twenty dollars
for a single one. It is the same with being overweight. Until you are consumed with pain, you will continue to let the doughnuts or the French fries
control you, unless your brain works right and you are able to stay focused
on what's motivating you to get healthy.

The pain and consequences that inspire change are different for each person. In your case, your weight problem may be causing health conditions, self-loathing, relationship troubles, or career roadblocks. In addition, everybody's threshold for pain is different. For example, one person who is 20 pounds overweight might hear a single unkind comment about their size or a warning from their doctor and decide to take action. Another individual may balloon up to more than 500 pounds and have endured years of insults and serious health problems before taking that first step to weight loss.

GET SMART TO GET THINNER

"My knee was causing me problems, and I realized that if I didn't get rid of the extra weight, it would make my knee worse."

—Curt

For you to change, you need to understand why you are uncomfortable. Only then can you make the decision to change your brain so you can break free from your unhealthy behavior.

How has being overweight or unhealthy caused you pain? Write it down here or use a separate sheet of paper. Don't leave anything out no matter how trivial you may believe it to be. When you have your list, mark the things that have been the most hurtful, that brought you the most shame, or that you want to make sure you never experience again.

THE PAIN I HAVE FELT FROM BEING OVERWEIGHT

_____

_____

_____

_____

_____

_____

Hope Is Healing

Hope is what makes you believe that you can change and that your weight, and your life, will be better if you succeed in giving up your bad habits. Without it, you will never take that first step to change or be able to follow a program long enough to create lasting weight loss.

How do you find that hope? Sometimes it can be generated by someone you respect—a teacher, a pastor, a doctor, or an author. My hope is that this book and the many success stories it contains will infuse you with hope so you will stick with the Amen Solution and boost your brain to be thinner, smarter, and happier. I have seen this program work for so many people, and I know it can work for you too.

What are the things that fill you with hope? Create a list of people, books, songs, and anything else that makes you feel hopeful about your ability to change your ways.

MY HOPE LIST

_____

_____

_____

_____

_____

Find Something You Love More Than Food—Starting with Your Brain

Finding the motivation to take that first step is one thing. Staying motivated throughout your weight-loss journey is another. One of the keys to staying motivated is finding something you can be passionate about that keeps you feeling energized and excited. Of course, this does *not* mean a passion for double-bacon cheeseburgers. Many people mistake an addiction to food for passion. You have to be careful not to get too much pleasure from your passions, or your brain's reward system could hijack your brain (more on this in chapter 6).

You need to fall in love with something other than the foods that are making you fat and unhappy, something that serves you. For me, falling in love with my brain was a critical step. Over the years I have personally had

---

GET SMART TO GET THINNER

"The Amen Solution starts with the brain! No other weight-loss program I've tried talks about the brain! I wish I would have learned this years ago."

—Jackson

ten brain SPECT, or single photon emission computed tomography, scans to check on the health of my own brain. SPECT is one of the main brain imaging studies we do at the Amen Clinics. It is a nuclear medicine study that looks at blood flow and activity patterns in the brain.

Looking back, my earliest scan, taken when I was thirty-seven, showed a toxic, bumpy appearance that was definitely not consistent with great brain function. See the scans below. All my life I have been someone who rarely drank alcohol, never smoked, and never used an illegal drug. Then why did my brain look so bad? Before I understood about brain health, I had many bad brain habits. I ate lots of fast food, lived on diet sodas, would often get by on four or five hours of sleep at night. In addition, I worked like a nut, didn't exercise much, and carried an extra 20–30 pounds that I had trouble losing.

My last scan, at age fifty-two, looks healthier and much younger than my first scan, even though brains typically become less active with age. Why? Seeing other people's scans, I developed "brain envy" and wanted mine to be

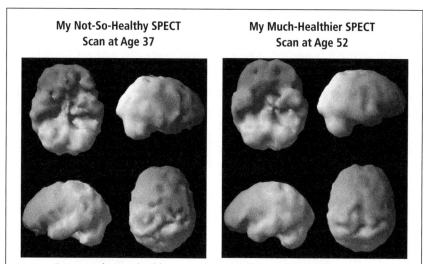

My Not-So-Healthy SPECT Scan at Age 37	My Much-Healthier SPECT Scan at Age 52
Bumpy and not so healthy	Fuller, overall healthier appearance

SPECT is a nuclear medicine study that looks at blood flow and activity patterns. The scan at the top left is looking at the undersurface of the brain. The scan at the bottom right is looking down from the top. The other two views look at the brain from the sides. These are called surface scans because they are looking at the outside surface of the brain. Here we are looking at the top 45 percent of brain activity. Anything below that level shows up as a hole or a dent, which means low areas of activity. Notice that my brain scan at age fifty-two looks fuller and less wrinkled. It looks healthier, even though brains usually look less active with age.

better. As I learned about brain health, I put into practice what I am teaching you and preached to my patients. Loving your brain is the first step toward creating a brain healthy life and getting to the weight you want.

Like me, you need to fall in love with your own brain. Practically, this means having the desire to take great care of it, protecting it, nourishing it, and focusing on its health. Here are four reasons why you need to love your brain.

THE BRAIN IS INVOLVED IN EVERYTHING YOU DO.

At every moment of every day of your life, your brain heavily influences how you think, feel, act, and interact with others. It is your brain that pushes you away from the table telling you that you have had enough, and it is your brain that gives you permission to have the second piece of cake, making you look and feel like a blob.

WHEN YOUR BRAIN WORKS RIGHT, YOU WORK RIGHT.

When your brain is healthy, it makes it much easier to make the right decisions when it comes to eating, drinking, and exercising. A healthy brain gets you to bed at a reasonable time so that you can get the rest you need and manages the stress in your life so you don't feel the need to turn to food for solace.

WHEN YOUR BRAIN IS TROUBLED, YOU HAVE TROUBLE IN YOUR LIFE.

When your brain is troubled, it creates trouble in every aspect of your life. It is harder to follow a healthy diet and exercise program and makes you more likely to fall into bad habits like drinking, smoking, and binge eating.

YOU CAN CHANGE YOUR BRAIN AND ENHANCE YOUR LIFE!

The best thing about your brain is that it can change. Even if you haven't been treating your brain with TLC, you can make it better! By avoiding bad brain habits and adopting as many good brain habits as possible, you can improve brain function and reduce your weight.

To stay motivated, find other passions too. What are the things that interest you in life? Cars? Sports (without head injury risk, of course)? Writing?

Reading? Animals? Your kids? Get a piece of paper and write down all the things you love or that make you happy. If you don't zero in on something right away, don't get discouraged. Give yourself some time. You may not discover your true passion until your brain is optimized.

NON-FOOD THINGS I LOVE

_____

_____

_____

_____

_____

The Amen Solution All-Stars: Ray and Nancy

Ray White came to see us as part of our NFL study. He played linebacker for the San Diego Chargers in the early 1970s. One of Ray's motivations for participating in our study was that his wife, Nancy, had been recently diagnosed with frontal temporal lobe dementia. When we evaluated Ray, he showed evidence of brain trauma (as did almost all of our retired players), plus he was overweight. Nancy's scans were a disaster. She had severe decreased activity in the front part of her brain, consistent with the diagnosis of frontal temporal lobe dementia.

The feedback session, in which I showed them their scans, was very emotional for Ray and Nancy—and for me too. We had experience already that showed we could help Ray. But there is no known effective treatment for frontal temporal lobe dementia. My bias with cases like Nancy's is to do everything we can to try to slow or reverse the dementia process. Certainly, it does not always work. In this case, I told Ray and Nancy that it was critical to immediately get on a brain healthy program, eat right, stop drinking alcohol, take their supplements, exercise, and I recommended hyperbaric oxygen treatment and neurofeedback for Nancy. I also told Ray he needed to start losing weight. His BMI was 31.

Ten weeks later I saw them back for their first follow-up visit. This visit was also emotional but in a much more positive way. Nancy had followed through on the recommendations for eating right, taking her supplements, eliminating alcohol, and she had forty hyperbaric oxygen sessions and sixteen neurofeedback sessions. She had significantly improved. Her memory

Nancy: Frontal Temporal Lobe Dementia

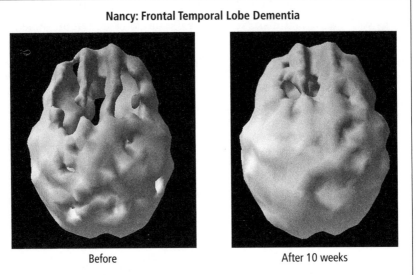

Before   After 10 weeks

Brain SPECT study showing blood flow and activity patterns. This view is looking down from the top, where the front part of the brain is at the top of the scan and the back part of the brain is at the bottom. The holes are areas of low activity. Notice the dramatic improvement in the front part of her brain.

and cognitive function were better, her personal grooming had improved, and she was doing better taking care of their home. Ray joked that we had to slow down, because soon enough she would be smarter than him. Nancy's follow up SPECT study showed dramatic improvement (see above). In addition, Ray had lost 30 pounds! He said his motivation was to help his wife. If he did everything we suggested, then she would too. They would do it as a couple. Sometimes motivation is about love. Ray loved Nancy.

Get in Touch with Your Spiritual Side

This may seem like an odd recommendation to some of you. What does spirituality have to do with motivating yourself to stop overeating? You may be surprised to discover that it can play a very important role in changing your behavior. First, let me explain that when I talk about spirituality here, I am not necessarily talking about organized religion, although that can be very helpful for some people. Think of spirituality in the broader sense of feeling connected to something greater than yourself, feeling connected to a higher power, feeling connected to the earth, feeling connected to past generations, feeling connected to future generations, feeling connected to your community, or feeling connected to a weight-loss support group.

Having a sense of belonging can be an important step in your journey to get healthy. Many people believe that their weight problems affect no one but themselves. Wrong! Being overweight or obese can impact your family, your friends, your community, and even your place of employment. Being overweight and miserable can take a terrible toll on your marriage. You are more likely to die an early death—remember, obesity is the third most common preventable cause of death—and leave your spouse alone. Your children may follow in your overeating footsteps and develop type 2 diabetes or other health problems. One of my childhood friends is very overweight. His oldest son is as well. It is clear that the son adopted his dad's bad eating habits, which has made it very hard for him to change, which in turn will affect his own children, and so on. Also, you may get sick and have to go on work disability, adding extra costs for your employer and our society.

GET SMART TO GET THINNER

"Writing in this fantastic *Daily Journal* is holding me very accountable for my feelings, thoughts, intentions, and food choices."

—Victoria

Feeling connected, rather than alone and isolated, instills a sense of accountability. When you feel accountable to a higher power, to your society, to your family, or to the others in your group, your actions matter, and it becomes important to get healthy not only for your own good but also for theirs. The people in our weight-loss groups have said that belonging to the group made them feel a greater sense of accountability. "I knew they were all counting on me," said one participant. "I didn't want to let them down."

There are three specific brain-based reasons why our in-person and online group programs are so successful. It is because it provides the three *F*s: frontal lobes, family and friends (limbic bonding), and fear.

FRONTAL LOBES (RULES)

The front part of your brain, the prefrontal cortex, is involved with executive functions, such as rule-oriented behavior and internal supervision. It is the little voice in your head that helps you decide between right and wrong, between the apple and the apple pie. The Amen Solution gives you a very clear set of guidelines and rules. It gives you structure. I often say it gives people an extra frontal lobe to help supervise their lives.

FAMILY AND FRIENDS (LIMBIC BONDING)

People who are struggling with weight gain often do not feel a strong connection to anything or anyone. You may not be fully engaged in your life, and you may think you must lose the weight before you can really start living your life. You may be familiar with these kinds of thoughts: "I want to lose 20 pounds before I start dating again" or "I don't fit in with any of the girls at work—they're all skinny." But the human brain needs bonding in order to achieve optimal functioning. Our in-person and online weight loss groups take on the role of a family-and-friends support group. This feeds the limbic area of the brain, which is involved in motivation and mood control.

FEAR (WHAT YOU DO HAS CONSEQUENCES)

Some people, me included, need fear to spur action. In this program, I introduce you to the fact that being overweight or obese is not only bad for your physical health, but it is also bad for your brain! (See the section Being Fat Is Bad for Your Brain, which follows.) And I have the brain scans to show you just how damaging the consequences of obesity can be. Brain imaging is very powerful and can strike fear in even the most complacent or stubborn people. I have seen it happen thousands of times. I am hoping that the many brain scans in this book will induce some anxiety in you about your weight. A little anxiety can be a great motivator! Anxiety mixed with frontal lobe help and limbic bonding is the perfect combination for people who want to lose weight.

Being Fat Is Bad for Your Brain

If you need more compelling evidence to motivate you to change, consider that in 2010 an expert panel declared, "The obesity epidemic is the single biggest threat to public health in this century." I would add that obesity is one of the biggest threats to brain health. Being overweight or obese is terrible for brain function. That, at least, is the gloomy conclusion of several recent studies, including the one I mentioned in the introduction from the University of Pittsburgh showing that people who are overweight or obese have smaller brains that look older than they really are.

- One long-term study of more than sixty-five hundred people in northern California found that those who were fat around the middle at age forty were more likely to succumb to dementia in their seventies.

- A 2010 study in the *Annals of Neurology* found that among healthy middle-aged people, the higher your BMI, and specifically the more belly fat you have, the less total brain volume you have.

- A long-term study in Sweden found that compared with thinner people, those who were overweight in their forties experienced a more rapid and more pronounced decline in brain function over the next several decades.

- A 2010 study analyzing data from 8,745 postmenopausal women found that the fatter a woman is, the worse her cognitive function and the more likely she is to have memory loss.

Consistent with this, the brains of obese people often show signs of damage. One study of sixty healthy young adults (in their twenties and thirties) found that the fatter members of the group had significantly lower gray-matter densities in several brain regions, including those involved in the perception of taste and the regulation of eating behavior. A study of 114 middle-aged people (aged between forty and sixty-six) found that the obese tended to have smaller, more atrophied brains than thinner people; other studies have found similar results.

GET SMART TO GET THINNER

"I attended a weight-loss lecture from another diet program, and I almost laughed out loud. It was like visiting a prekindergarten school after experiencing and attending the graduate school of the Amen Solution."

—Paul

Brains usually atrophy with age, but being obese appears to accelerate the process. This is bad news—pronounced brain atrophy is a feature of dementia. Why being overweight should affect the brain in this way is not clear, although a host of culprits have been suggested. A paper published in *Proceedings of the National Academy of Sciences* has identified a gene that seems to be involved. FTO, as the gene is known, appears to play a role in both body weight and brain function. This gene comes in different versions; one version—let's call it "troublesome"—appears to predispose people to obesity. Individuals with two copies of the troublesome version tend to be fatter than those with only one copy of it, who in turn tend to be fatter than those with two copies of the "regular" version. Now the troublesome form has been linked to atrophy in several regions of the brain, including the frontal lobes, though how and why it has this effect remains unknown.

Yet your genes are not your destiny. I took a test from a genetic testing company that reported I had a 65 percent chance of being overweight. My genes say I am supposed to be fat and indeed I have many overweight family members. But genes are not the whole story. It also has to do with how much you eat and other habits.

Obesity exacerbates problems like sleep apnea, which can result in the brain being starved of oxygen; this can lead to brain damage. Obesity often goes along with high blood pressure, heart disease, and diabetes, all of which are bad for the brain in their own right. Indeed, one study has shown that if, in middle age, you are obese and have high blood pressure, the two problems gang up on you, increasing the chances of your getting dementia in old age more than either one would do on its own.

Fat tissue itself is a problem. Fat cells secrete substances called cytokines that cause inflammation. Chronic inflammation of the brain, which is often found in the obese, impairs learning and memory and is a feature of depression and Alzheimer's. Diet also plays a role. Studies in mice have shown that eating a very high-fat diet increases brain inflammation and disrupts brain function. And the onset of brain decay may itself play a part. Since the regions of the brain most affected by obesity appear to be those involved in self-control and the regulation of appetite, erosion of these abilities may lead to greater obesity, which may lead to more rapid brain erosion, in a downward spiral.

Whatever the causes, the implications are grave. In the United States today, about one-third of adults are obese. At the same time, dementia is already one of the most costly and devastating health problems of old age. The possibility that obesity today will lead to higher rates of dementia in the future is, therefore, deeply alarming.

The obvious question is: can obesity-associated brain damage be reversed? I am convinced that it can, and have seen enhanced brain function in my practice for twenty years. Science has already shown that brain shrinkage can be reversed. A 2010 study from a research team at the Columbia University for Eating Disorders showed that women with anorexia have less gray-matter volume than healthy-weight women. The longer the women had been in the clutches of the illness, the greater the shrinkage. The researchers found that after the women increased their weight, brain volume was restored. If brain volume can be enhanced when the severely under-weight reach a healthy weight, it makes sense that obese people who achieve a healthy weight can also reverse brain shrinkage.

But now would be the time to start. Those two old friends, a healthful diet and plenty of exercise, have repeatedly been shown to protect the brain. Foods like oily fishes and organic blueberries have been shown to stimulate the growth of new neurons, for example. Moreover, one study found that dieting reversed some of the changes to brain structure found among the obese. Whether you are fat or thin, young or old, the best hope you have of guarding your brain is to eat well and exercise. Has anyone seen my running shoes?

Stay Focused by Using Your Frontal Lobes

To stay focused on losing the love handles, you have to strengthen your frontal lobes. The front half of the frontal lobes is called the prefrontal cortex, which is involved with attention, planning, judgment, impulse control, and follow-through. These are all critical components for weight-loss success, so you can do the following.

- Pay attention to what you eat (no mindless eating!).
- Plan meals and snacks so you don't get stuck without any brain healthy options, and plan how you are going to squeeze physical activity into your day.
- Make the best decisions throughout the day.
- Say no when the server brings the dessert tray to your table and asks if you saved room for the mocha mud pie.
- Follow through on your plans rather than just thinking about them.

One of the best ways to boost your prefrontal cortex power is to set goals. I recommend you set SMART goals. Setting the right kind of goals can help you achieve those goals and reduce the risk of failure. SMART goals are:

- Specific
- Measurable
- Attainable
- Realistic
- Timely

SPECIFIC

You have a better chance of achieving a specific goal rather than a vague goal. For example, "Eat oatmeal with organic blueberries for breakfast instead of fast food" is a better goal than "Eat better."

MEASURABLE

When you can measure your goals, it is easier to know if you are on the right path to achieving them, and measuring lets you know when you have reached your goal. For example, "Go to the gym four times a week for thirty minutes each session" is a better goal than "Get in shape."

ATTAINABLE

Set short-term goals that you are capable of achieving. These short-term goals will help keep you motivated toward your long-term goals. Setting goals that are too lofty or long-term can be demotivating. For example, "Lose 100 pounds in one year" sounds impossible. "Lose 2 pounds a week" doesn't sound so hard, but it will get you to that bigger goal. When you give yourself attainable short-term goals, it makes it easier for you to believe in your ability to change. To effect change, you must believe in your ability to make it happen. If you don't believe, you'll never do it.

REALISTIC

Goals that are unrealistic set you up to feel like a failure. For example, "Run a marathon next month" may be completely unrealistic if you have never run a single mile in your life. A realistic goal is one that you are both willing and able to achieve. If you really do want to participate in a race, your goal might be "Walk or run a 5K in three months." This gives you time to practice so you won't injure yourself and improves your chances of successfully completing the event.

TIMELY

Goals that have no timeframe lack urgency. Set a specific timeframe, such as "by March 15" or "starting today" to force you into action.

One-Page Miracle

One of the most powerful yet simple exercises I have designed is called the One-Page Miracle. It will help guide nearly all of your thoughts, words, and actions. It is a "miracle" because I've seen this exercise quickly focus and change many people's lives. It is particularly effective for people who want to lose weight because it makes you focus on what is truly important to you and forces you to think about long-term goals rather than just the immediate gratification that comes from mindless eating or bingeing.

As you will see, this exercise asks you to include your hopes and dreams for four specific areas—biological, psychological, social, and spiritual. That is because being overweight isn't simply an eating problem. There can be biological factors, psychological reasons, social issues, and spiritual troubles contributing to your weight problem, and you need to address all four areas if you are going to break free from the chains that are keeping you fat.

DIRECTIONS

Make copies of "My One-Page Miracle" on page 54 use the One-Page Miracle maker on our website, or use a sheet of paper and clearly write out a rough draft of your major goals for the four pillars of weight loss: biological, psychological, social, and spiritual. If you are using a piece of paper, include the subcategories "Brain Health," "Physical Health," "Eating," "Weight," and "Exercise" under the heading "Biological." Under the heading "Psychological," write "Emotional Health" and "Thinking Patterns." Under the heading "Social," include "Relationships," "Children," "Support," and "Work/ Money." Under the heading "Spiritual," write "Spirituality," "Passions," and "Meaning."

Next to each subheading succinctly write out what's important to you in that area; write what you want, not what you don't want. Be positive and use the first person. Write what you want with confidence and the expectation that you will make it happen. Remember to make your goals SMART (specific, measurable, attainable, realistic, and timely). Keep the paper with you so that you can work on it over several days or weeks.

After you finish with the initial draft (you'll want to update it frequently), place this piece of paper where you can see it every day, such as on your refrigerator, by your bedside, or on the bathroom mirror. In that way, every day you focus your eyes on what's important to you. This makes it easier to match your behavior to what you want. Your life becomes more conscious and you spend your energy on goals that are important to you.

Here is an example I did with one of my obese patients who was suffering from depression. Zoe, thirty-one, started binge eating in high school when her boyfriend dumped her. That started a pattern of bingeing whenever she felt sad or stressed, like when she didn't get chosen by the sorority she had pledged and when she got passed over for a promotion at work. Even though she had gained more than 60 pounds since high school and couldn't look at herself in the mirror, she couldn't stop her secret bingeing. She avoided dating because she didn't see how any man could find her attractive, and she was so depressed about her weight that she had stopped participating in activities she used to enjoy, like playing the piano.

Zoe's brain SPECT scans showed too much activity in the deep limbic system, which is involved with mood, motivation, and appetite. They also revealed an overactive anterior cingulate gyrus, which is common in people who get stuck on thoughts, such as thoughts about food. It is also common in people with binge eating disorders.

After you look at the example, fill out the One-Page Miracle for yourself. If you have prefrontal cortex challenges, which are common in people with food addictions and overeating, this exercise will be very helpful for you. After you complete this exercise, put it up where you can see and read it every day. It is a great idea to start the day off each day by reading your One-Page Miracle to get focused on what really matters to you. Then before you do or say something, ask yourself if your potential behavior fits your goals.

ZOE'S ONE-PAGE MIRACLE

BIOLOGICAL—to be the healthiest I can be

    Brain health: To love my brain starting *today,* and before I do anything I will think about how it will affect the health of my brain.

    Physical health: To make an appointment with my doctor next week to check my important health numbers and to optimize anything that is out of whack.

    Eating: To throw out all the junk food in my kitchen *today* and start following the Amen Clinics Seven Rules for Brain Healthy Eating.

    Weight: To lose 1 pound per week for the next twenty weeks, then maintain it by following the steps in this program.

    Exercise: To do thirty minutes of fast walking four times a week.

PSYCHOLOGICAL—to love myself, respect myself, and be forgiving of myself

    Emotional health: To exercise, take fish oil, and SAMe to help deal with my depression and, if I still need help, to see a mental health professional, plus to practice healthier ways to deal with stress.

    Thinking patterns: To kill the ANTs (automatic negative thoughts), to focus on the positive, to believe in myself, and to be grateful every day.

SOCIAL—to be connected to those I love and to develop a strong support group

    Relationships: To open myself up to dating, and maybe spend some time online at reputable dating sites.

    Children: No children now, but when I do have kids, I want to be a great role model.

    Support: To join an online weight-loss community this week.

    Work/Money: To feel more confident about myself so I can apply for the outside sales job at work.

SPIRITUAL—To feel connected to a higher power and others

    Spirituality: To meditate daily

    Passions: To start playing the piano again by taking piano lessons once a week

    Meaning: To make a difference in someone else's life today

MY ONE-PAGE MIRACLE

What Do I Want? What Am I Doing to Make It Happen?

BIOLOGICAL

Brain health: _____

Physical health: _____

Eating: _____

Weight: _____

Exercise: _____

PSYCHOLOGICAL

Emotional health: _____

Thinking patterns: _____

SOCIAL

Relationships: _____

Children: _____

Support: _____

Work/Money: _____

SPIRITUAL

Spirituality: _____

Passions: _____

Meaning: _____

3

EAT RIGHT TO THINK RIGHT
AND KEEP TRACK OF WHAT YOU EAT

GET THINNER, SMARTER, AND HAPPIER

Whenever I meet with young people to talk about brain healthy nutrition, I ask them this: If you could have any car in the world, what would it be? A Ferrari? A Bentley? A Corvette? An Aston Martin? Usually, Ferrari leads the list. Whichever one is your dream car, I continue, I want you to imagine it with all of your senses. See the color, maybe bright red? See the leather seats, maybe black or camel color? Smell the fresh leather. See the car in your garage, new and perfect.

Now imagine someone coming into your garage and putting salt into the gas tank. How would you feel? What would you think? What would you do to that person? Many people, more guys than girls, get angry and say that they would hurt the person who ruined their special car.

Why? I ask them. Isn't that exactly what you to do yourself whenever you eat something that is bad for you, with excessive sugar, bad fat, or too much salt? Your body and brain are much more precious than any car could ever be! But you treat yourself with such disrespect; soon your body may break down like the car with salt in the gas tank. That's exactly the point of this chapter.

Just like a great car needs high-octane gasoline to keep its engine running at its best, your brain and body need premium fuel for optimal function. It's the fuel that you eat and drink that drives your brain and body to be thinner, smarter, and happier or fatter, dumber, and depressed. Nutrition makes a dramatic difference in brain and body health.

If you fuel your brain and body with brain healthy foods, it will help you be trim, vibrant, happy, and focused. Fuel up on junk food, and it can make you plump, sluggish, sad, and stupid. The choice seems obvious. And logically every one of us would choose the premium fuel. But our society and eating habits have changed so drastically that many of us no longer recognize which foods are good for us and which ones are disasters. When you pull up to any modern-day brain-body fueling station—grocery stores, restaurants, delis, sporting event vendors, convenience stores, and so on—you don't get to choose between just "premium" and "regular." You have thousands of choices, many of which might seem healthy but actually aren't.

To help you navigate your way to the best options that will help you slim down, boost your cognitive function, and lift your mood, I have come up with the Amen Clinics Seven Rules for Brain Healthy Eating. These rules apply to everybody, regardless of your brain type. You will learn more about specific eating plans based on brain type in chapter 4.

RULE 1. THINK HIGH-QUALITY CALORIES IN VERSUS HIGH-QUALITY ENERGY OUT.

Don't let anyone tell you that calories don't count. They absolutely do. But it is not as simple as calories in versus calories out. I admit that I used to think that as long as I stayed within a certain calorie range, my weight would be fine. But I was wrong.

GET SMART TO GET THINNER

"For the first time in my life, I am aware of the food I eat—both quality *and* quantity."

—Gina

You have to focus on eating "high-quality calories." That means eating the apple instead of the apple pie à la mode, the almonds instead of the Almond Roca, and the steel-cut organic oatmeal instead of the oatmeal cookie.

The research about calories is very clear. If you eat more calories than you need, you will be fatter, sicker, and less productive. In a famous study involving rhesus monkeys, researchers followed a large group of monkeys for twenty years. One group ate all the food they wanted; the other group ate 30 percent less. The monkeys who ate anything they wanted were three times more likely to suffer from cancer, heart disease, and diabetes. Plus, researchers saw significant shrinkage in the important decision-making areas of their brains. Over the two decades of the study half of the all-you-can-eat monkeys died while only 20 percent of the restricted-calorie monkeys died.

Many diet programs today have discarded the traditional concept of calorie reduction. Instead, they insist that you need to eat a specific ratio of protein, carbohydrates, and fats in order to lose weight. Not so, according to a recent study in the *New England Journal of Medicine* conducted at the Harvard School of Public Health and Brigham and Women's Hospital. This study found that calorie reduction—regardless of the percentage of fats, carbohydrates, or proteins in a diet—is what leads to weight loss. For this study, the researchers enlisted 811 overweight individuals and assigned them to one of the following four diets:

- 20 percent fat, 15 percent protein, 65 percent carbohydrates
- 20 percent fat, 25 percent protein, 55 percent carbohydrates
- 40 percent fat, 15 percent protein, 45 percent carbohydrates
- 40 percent fat, 25 percent protein, 35 percent carbohydrates

At the conclusion of the two-year study, all four groups had achieved a similar weight loss of an average of nearly nine pounds.

Restricting calories does *not* mean starving yourself. Crash dieting isn't doing your brain or body any favors. Extremely low calorie intake is associated with a lack of nutrients, which can deprive your brain and body of the fuel needed for optimal performance. Plus, this way of eating is not sustainable in the long run. It doesn't teach you how to eat right to maintain a healthy weight, so after you drop the pounds, you go back to your old bad habits and regain the weight. I'll bet many of you have been there, done that.

GET SMART TO GET THINNER

"I'm figuring out ways to get the flavors of the things I really like without all the calories. I loved banana bread. Now I eat a banana with a few walnuts and it's kind of like banana nut bread. I have stevia and cinnamon on apples and it's kind of like apple pie. It's so easy! But a year ago, if you had told me to do that I would have said you're crazy."

—Irene

Be a value spender. Think of calories like money. You only have a certain amount of calories you can spend each day in order to reach your goal weight, so you want to spend very wisely, or you will bankrupt your brain and body.

My wife says I am not a cheap person but rather a *value spender*. I hate wasting money. Once, I had a firm do work for our clinics, and even though their work was acceptable, I felt that they had overbilled me for the effort, so I avoided them in the future. I have this same attitude toward food. I hate wasting calories on foods that will drain my brain, make me fat, and leave me feeling sluggish.

If you are like me and you like to get a lot of bang for your buck, choose foods that offer the most *nutritional* value rather than wasting your precious calories on foods that cause brain fog and keep you fat. For example, one slice of strawberry cheesecake can cost you 730 calories, drain your brain, put you on an emotional roller coaster, and increase your appetite and cravings. On the other hand, a 400-calorie salad made of spinach, salmon, blueberries, apples, walnuts, and red bell peppers will supercharge your energy and make you smarter.

You have to realize that when I talk about being a value spender, I am not talking about those so-called value meals the fast-food restaurants offer. Most of them are actually robbing you of brain healthy nutrients and costing you far more in terms of your health and well-being. Cheap food may be the most expensive in terms of our long-term health. A 2010 study in the *FASEB Journal* shows that you need to kill the junk food—or it will kill you early. This study found that when mice consumed high levels of phosphates, found in soft drinks and many processed foods, it sped up the aging process and led to early death. Where's the value in that? Be a value spender when it comes to calories, or you will bankrupt your brain and body.

Know the calorie counts of the foods and beverages you are eating! U.S. health care reform legislation passed in 2010 requires large chain restaurants to post calorie counts on menus. Many eateries also make nutritional information available on their websites. Make it a practice to look up menus online *before* you go out so you know which menu items will give you the most nutritional value for the calorie cost. You can also find out how many calories are in hundreds of foods in appendix C or using the nutrition tools on our website.

GET SMART TO GET THINNER

"If I'm going to splurge on something, I figure out how to make it work *within* my calorie budget."

—Pamela

A colleague of mine was recently invited to a chain restaurant that is famous for its pizza. She knew it might be difficult to find something on the menu that was light on calories but high in brain healthy nutrients, so she spent a few minutes analyzing the nutritional information online. She found a salad (a half order) that was loaded with grilled vegetables and salmon, packed with protein and fiber, and low in saturated fat for about 600 calories. If she hadn't done her homework, she could have ended up ordering a salad that sounded healthy but weighed in at more than 1,500 calories.

A lot of my patients ask me if it is possible to eat fast food while watching their calorie intake. The answer is yes. Many fast-food restaurants are adding healthier, low-calorie fare to their menu options. To help you make better choices at fast-food restaurants, here is a chart of an entire day's meals (breakfast, lunch, afternoon snack, dinner, and dessert) with calorie busters to avoid and lighter options that get the green light.

	JUST SAY NO!	ORDER THIS INSTEAD!
	BREAKFAST	
Burger King:	Double Croissan'wich with double sausage	Breakfast Muffin Sandwich
	Cini-minis	BK Fresh Apple Fries
	Mocha BK Joe iced coffee	BK Joe Decaf (small)
Total:	**1,440 calories**	**475 calories**
	LUNCH	
Taco Bell:	Chicken Ranch Taco Salad	2 Fresco Ranchero Chicken Soft Tacos
	Volcano Nachos	Pintos 'n Cheese
	Lipton raspberry iced tea (40 oz.)	Water
Total:	**2,310 calories**	**510 calories**
	AFTERNOON SNACK	
Jack in the Box:	Sampler Trio (2 egg rolls, 3 mozzarella cheese sticks, 3 stuffed jalapenos)	Fruit Cup
	794 calories	**54 calories**

	JUST SAY NO!	ORDER THIS INSTEAD!
	DINNER	
Carl's Jr.:	Double Western Bacon Cheeseburger	Charbroiled BBQ Chicken burger
	Chili Cheese Fries	Garden Side Salad (with low-fat balsamic)
	Banana Chocolate Chip Hand-Scooped Ice Cream Shake	Water
Total:	**2,720 calories**	**465 calories**
	DESSERT	
McDonald's:	3 chocolate chip cookies	Snack Size Fruit and Walnut Salad
Total:	**480 calories**	**210 calories**
Grand total for the day:	**7,744 calories**	**1,714 calories**

If calorie counts are not listed on the menu, ask! Use your brain, be smart, and do not let other people make you fat and unhappy. Take control of your eating rather than letting a restaurant or ballpark vendor dictate how many calories you eat.

GET SMART TO GET THINNER

"Measuring my food opened up a whole new world of self-abuse. I had no idea how much I was eating."

—Reggie

At the grocery store, *read the nutrition labels!* Many products that are marketed as "healthy" are in reality high-calorie, low-nutrient losers. Be sure to check the serving size on the labels. If you are like most Americans, your idea of a serving size is probably very different from the one listed. You might look at a box of bran cereal that says 100 calories per serving and think that's a great value. But how much of it are you really eating? I was shocked when I actually measured out the suggested serving size of a cup of cereal. I had been eating at least twice that much but thinking I was only eating 100 calories.

This is why it is absolutely critical that you get a food scale, measuring cups, and measuring spoons and measure and weigh *everything* you eat. This takes the guesswork out of counting calories and makes you be honest with yourself about how much you are eating. I can tell you that among our weight-loss group participants, the ones who buy a food scale and measure their food are typically the most successful.

Know how many calories a day you need to eat to either maintain your weight or lose weight. The average active fifty-year-old man needs about 2,200 calories a day to maintain his weight, and the average fifty-year-old woman needs about 1,800 calories. You can find calorie calculators on our website to help you determine your individual calorie needs.

Here is an example from Sherri, one of our weight-loss group participants. She used our online calorie calculator to determine how many calories she needed to maintain her current weight (at the debut of the program).

- Height: 5'5"
- Weight: 168 pounds
- Gender: female
- Age: 40
- Activity lifestyle: sedentary
- Result: She needed a total of 1,804 calories to maintain her current weight.

With this information, Sherri was then able to figure out how many calories she needs to eat in order to lose 1 pound per week. To lose one pound per week, you need to reduce your daily intake by 500 calories below your requirements. That is based on the fact that 1 pound of fat contains approximately 3,500 calories, so to lose 1 pound a week, you need to consume approximately 3,500 fewer calories per week. Divide 3,500 by seven days, and you get 500 calories per day. I recommend you use a combination of diet and exercise to reduce your intake by 500 calories. For example, eat 200 fewer calories and burn an additional 300 calories through exercise. So for Sherri, she needs to reduce her calorie intake to 1,604 calories a day, with 300 calories of exercise, in order to lose 1 pound per week. Without exercise she needs to eat 1,304 calories a day.

Knowing your daily calorie allowance is only part of the weight-loss equation. You also need to know how many calories a day you actually put in your body. Keep a daily food journal (more on journaling later in this chapter) just like you keep a checkbook. Start the day with the number of calories you can spend, and write down *everything* you eat and drink throughout the day. That includes the handful of M&M's you grabbed from the receptionist's desk and the sweetened iced tea you had with lunch. This one strategy made a huge difference for me. When I actually wrote down everything I ate for a month, it caused me to stop lying to myself about my calories.

One of our NFL players wrote that when he started counting his calories, it opened up a new world of self-abuse that he was completely unaware of.

"High-quality energy out" means you need to expend energy and rev up your metabolism in healthy ways. Exercise, new learning, and green tea help. You will learn much more about workouts for your brain and body in chapter 7. As for green tea, numerous studies have found that the catechins found in green tea, such as epigallocatechin gallate, have a positive effect on metabolism, BMI, weight loss, waist circumference, and weight management.

When you are desperate to lose the love handles or the muffin top, you may be tempted to try unhealthy methods to expend more energy. Energy boosters to avoid include diet pills, sugary caffeinated energy drinks, too much coffee (green tea has half the caffeine as coffee), caffeinated sodas, smoking, and excessive exercise.

RULE 2. DRINK PLENTY OF WATER AND NOT TOO MANY OF YOUR CALORIES.

Did you know that your brain is 80 percent water? Anything that dehydrates it, such as too much caffeine or much alcohol, decreases your thinking and impairs your judgment. Proper hydration is one of the keys to weight loss! Since the hunger and thirst centers sit right next to each other in the brain, many times when we think we are hungry, we are really just dehydrated. So we mistake the thirst signal for a food signal!

To be properly hydrated, drink at least half your body weight in ounces. If you weigh 200 pounds, then you need to drink about 100 ounces of water a day. That is about three quarts. Go to the store and buy a quart (32 ounces) bottle of water and fill it up three times a day. Start drinking it in the morning and bring your bottle with you throughout the day. In no time, you will figure out how to fit three quarts of water into your daily routine.

You are what you drink. Guzzling sugar-filled, fat-filled sodas, coffee treats, cocktails, sports drinks, fruit juices, and whole milk throughout the day can make you fat and sabotage your efforts to slim down. Just look at the approximate calorie counts for some of America's favorite beverages. The counts are for 12 ounces of each beverage so you can compare which ones are the most caloric. It may surprise you.

BEVERAGE CALORIE COUNTS

12 ounces ginger ale	120 calories
12 ounces orange juice	135 calories
12 ounces grapefruit juice	140 calories
12 ounces cola	150 calories
12 ounces Red Bull	165 calories
12 ounces cranberry juice	200 calories
12 ounces whole milk	215 calories

DON'T DRINK THESE CALORIE HOGS

Starbucks Venti Peppermint White Chocolate Mocha with whole milk and whipped cream	700 calories
Long Island iced tea	780 calories
Margarita	740 calories
McDonald's Chocolate McCafé Shake (15.8 ounces)	880 calories
Smoothie King's The Hulk Strawberry (40 ounces)	2,070 calories

The first step to limiting liquid calories is becoming aware of exactly how many you are drinking. On your daily food journal, be sure to include everything you drink throughout the day, including those free refills of soda and coffee with cream and sugar—the calories still count even if they are consumed in the same cup at the same sitting.

GET SMART TO GET THINNER

"I stopped drinking wine with dinner every night and lost 23 pounds and have so much more energy. But then I went on vacation and split a bottle of wine each night with my wife. I felt poisoned and had no energy. When I returned home, I cut out the wine again and felt so much better."

—Thomas

A growing body of evidence shows a strong connection between sugar-laden beverages and weight gain. Take the Harvard Nurses' Health Study, for example, which tracked more than fifty thousand women over an eight-year period. In this large-scale study, researchers found that women who increased their consumption of sugar-sweetened beverages during the eight years packed on a significant amount of weight while women who reduced their consumption experienced less weight gain.

Liquid calories are especially troublesome when you are trying to lose weight because they don't trigger the hormones in the brain that tell us we feel full. For example, researchers have found that the high-fructose corn syrup found in many sodas does not stimulate these hormones. Even highly caloric drinks like protein shakes don't satisfy hunger the way solid food does. This means that drinking all those extra liquid calories doesn't make you eat less food; it simply increases the total number of calories you consume.

Two studies testing the effects of beverage consumption on food intake: In one six-week study, researchers examined eighteen female and fifteen male volunteers and their lunch-eating habits in relation to beverage consumption. The foods they ate were the same each day, but meals were accompanied by a rotation of soda, diet soda, or water in two portion sizes: 12 ounces and 18 ounces. The researchers found that regardless of the size or beverage consumed, people ate the same amount of solid food. This translated into a bump in calories on the days sugary soda was served. In the other study, the researchers tracked forty-four women as they ate lunch accompanied by one of five beverages: water, diet soda, soda, orange juice, or 1% milk. Again, the amount of food calories consumed remained constant no matter which beverage was served.

More evidence comes from a study appearing in the *Journal of the American Dietetic Association*. In this trial, researchers gave twenty lean and twenty obese individuals one of the following—an apple, applesauce, or apple juice—either with a meal or as a snack. The results showed that drinking apple juice either with a meal or as a snack reduced hunger the least while eating an apple reduced hunger the most. These results were the same for both the lean and obese groups.

A study in the *International Journal of Obesity* showed that liquid calories contribute to more weight gain than eating jelly beans! In this trial, volunteers who ate the candy decreased the amount of other food calories they consumed while those who drank caloric beverages did not reduce their food intake.

GET SMART TO GET THINNER

"I was drinking wine with dinner every day. Just cutting that out cut a lot of calories."
—Melissa

The bottom line here is clear. Stop drinking beverages loaded with calories! Fortunately, reducing or eliminating liquid calories from your diet is one of the easiest and most effective ways to cut calories and shed extra pounds. Curbing your intake of liquid calories results in greater weight loss than cutting out food calories, according to a recent study that appeared in the *American Journal of Clinical Nutrition*. The study, which tracked the weight of 810 men and women, found that those who cut 100 liquid calories per day lost more weight than those who reduced their food intake by 100 calories. As you can see from the Beverage Calorie Counts list above, 100 calories is less than a single can of soda.

Learning to substitute brain healthy beverages—water, herbal teas, and unsweetened almond milk—for high-calorie drinks can put you on the fast track to weight loss. My favorite drink is water mixed with a little lemon juice and a little bit of the natural sweetener stevia. It tastes like lemonade, so I feel like I'm spoiling myself, and it has virtually no calories. Other drinks I like include: sparkling water with just a splash of cranberry juice, sparkling water with root-beer-flavored stevia, cinnamon tea with cinnamon-flavored stevia.

RULE 3. EAT HIGH-QUALITY LEAN PROTEIN THROUGHOUT THE DAY.

Protein helps balance your blood sugar and provides the necessary building blocks for brain health. Eating protein is important for anyone trying to lose weight, but it is especially critical for certain brain types. You will learn about these brain types in chapter 4.

Protein contains L-tyrosine, an amino acid that is important in the synthesis of brain neurotransmitters. Found in foods like meat, poultry, fish, and tofu, it is the precursor to dopamine, epinephrine, and norepinephrine, which are critical for balancing mood and energy. It is also helpful in the process of producing thyroid hormones, which are important in metabolism and energy production. Tyrosine supplementation has been shown to improve cognitive performance under periods of stress and fatigue. Stress tends to deplete the neurotransmitter norepinephrine, and tyrosine is the amino acid building block to replenish it.

Also found in protein is L-tryptophan, an amino acid building block for serotonin. L-tryptophan is found in meat, eggs, and milk. Increasing intake of L-tryptophan is very helpful for some people in stabilizing mood, improving mental clarity and sleep, and decreasing aggressiveness. Scientific evidence also shows that supplementation with L-tryptophan can help people lose weight.

Eating protein-rich foods like fish, chicken, and beef also provides the amino acid glutamine, which serves as the precursor to the neurotransmitter GABA. GABA is reported in the herbal literature to work in much the same way as antianxiety drugs and anticonvulsants. It helps stabilize nerve cells by decreasing their tendency to fire erratically or excessively. This means it has a calming effect for people who struggle with temper, irritability, and anxiety.

GET SMART TO GET THINNER

"Now I make sure to have a little protein with every meal and it helps balance my blood sugar and keep me from getting hungry."

—Jenna

Great sources of lean protein include fish, skinless turkey or chicken, beans, raw nuts, high-protein grains, and high-protein vegetables, such as broccoli and spinach. Quinoa (pronounced keen-wa) contains more protein than any other grain with 9 g per 1 cup of cooked quinoa. My wife, Tana, who is a nurse and the author of the *Change Your Brain, Change Your Body Cookbook,* often uses quinoa in soups, salads, and side dishes instead of rice, potatoes, or other grains to get a good protein boost.

It is especially important to eat protein at breakfast because it increases attention and focus, which we need for work or school. Eating carbohydrates boosts serotonin in the brain, which induces relaxation, and that makes you want to sleep through your morning meetings. In the United States, we have it backward. We tend to eat high-carbohydrate cereal, pancakes, or bagels for breakfast and a big steak for dinner. Doing the opposite may be a smarter move for your brain. I love the idea of using food to fuel your ability to focus or relax. If I need to work at night I will increase my protein. If it has been a stressful day I am more likely to eat pasta to calm my brain.

GET SMART TO GET THINNER

"I am seventy-one years old, and it is only recently that I realized I am addicted to sugar. I no longer eat sugar, and the cravings stopped. I eat healthy foods and have lost weight. I wish more doctors would talk to their patients about sugar addiction."

—Jen

RULE 4. EAT LOW-GLYCEMIC, HIGH-FIBER CARBOHYDRATES.

This means eat carbohydrates that do not spike your blood sugar and that are also high in fiber, such as whole grains, vegetables, and fruits like blueberries and apples. Carbohydrates are not the enemy. They are essential to your life. Bad carbohydrates are the enemy. These are carbohydrates that have been robbed of any nutritional value, such as simple sugars and refined carbohydrates.

Get to know the glycemic index. The glycemic index (GI) rates carbohydrates according to their effects on blood sugar. It is ranked on a scale from 1 to 100-plus. Low-glycemic foods have a low number (which means they do not spike your blood sugar, so they are generally healthier for you) and high-glycemic foods have a high number (which means they quickly elevate your blood sugar, so they are generally not as healthy for you).

Eating a diet that is filled with low-glycemic foods will lower your blood glucose levels, decrease cravings, and help with weight loss. The important concept to remember is that high blood sugar is bad for your brain and ultimately your waistline.

Be careful when going by GI to choose your foods. Some foods that are low glycemic aren't really healthy for you. For example, in the following list, you might notice that peanut M&M's have a GI of 33 whereas steel-cut oatmeal has a GI of about 52. Does this mean that it's better for you to eat peanut M&M's? No! Peanut M&M's are loaded with saturated fat, artificial food coloring, and other things that are not brain healthy. Steel-cut oatmeal is a high-fiber food that helps regulate your blood sugar for hours. Use your brain when choosing your food.

In general, vegetables, fruits, legumes, and nuts are the best low-GI options. A diet rich in low-GI foods not only helps you lose weight, it has also been found to help control diabetes, according to a 2010 review of the scientific literature in the *British Journal of Nutrition*. Be aware, however, that some foods that sound healthy actually have a high GI. For example, some fruits, like watermelon, have a high ranking. It is wise to consume more fruits on the low end of the spectrum. Similarly, some vegetables like potatoes and some high-fiber products like whole wheat bread are on the high end of the list. Eating smaller portions of these foods and combining them with lean proteins and healthy fats can reduce their impact on blood sugar levels.

The following list of foods and their GI is culled from numerous sources, including a 2008 review of nearly 2,500 individual food items by researchers at the Institute of Obesity, Nutrition and Exercise in Sydney, Australia. Make a copy of this list and keep it with you when you go grocery shopping.

GLYCEMIC INDEX

Low GI	55 and under
Medium GI	56–69
High GI	70–above

GLYCEMIC INDEX RATINGS

Grains	Glycemic Index
French baguette	83 ± 6
White bread	75 ± 2
Whole wheat bread	74 ± 2
White rice	72 ± 8
Bagel, white	69
Brown rice	66 ± 5
Couscous	65 ± 4
Hamburger bun	61
Basmati rice	57 ± 4
Quinoa	53
Spaghetti, white	49 ± 3
Pumpernickel bread	41
Barley, pearled	25 ± 2

Breakfast Foods	Glycemic Index
Scones	92 ± 8
Instant oatmeal	79 ± 3
Cornflakes	77
Waffles	76
Froot Loops	69 ± 9
Pancakes	66 ± 9
Kashi Seven Whole Grain Puffs	65 ± 10
Bran muffin	60
Blueberry muffin	59
Steel-cut oatmeal	52 ± 4
Kellogg's All-Bran	38

Fruit	Glycemic Index
(raw unless otherwise noted)	
Dates, dried	103 ± 21
Watermelon	80 ± 3
Pineapple	66 ± 7
Cantaloupe	65
Raisins	64 ± 11
Kiwi	58 ± 7
Mango	51 ± 5
Banana, overripe	48
Grapes	43
Nectarines	43 ± 6
Banana, underripe	42
Oranges	45 ± 4
Blueberries	40
Strawberries	40 ± 7
Plums	39
Pears	38 ± 2
Apples	36 ± 5
Apricots	34 ± 3
Peach	28
Grapefruit	25
Cherries	22

Vegetables	Glycemic Index
Instant mashed potato	87 ± 3
Baked potato	86 ± 6
Sweet potato	70 ± 6
French fries	64 ± 6
Sweet corn	52 ± 5
Peas	51 ± 6
Carrots, boiled	39 ± 4
Yam	35 ± 5
Artichoke	15
Asparagus	15
Broccoli	15
Cauliflower	15

Celery	15
Cucumber	15
Eggplant	15
Green beans	15
Lettuce	15
Peppers	15
Snow peas	15
Spinach	15
Squash	15
Tomatoes	15
Zucchini	15

Legumes and Nuts	Glycemic Index
Baked beans, canned	40 ± 3
Chickpeas	36 ± 5
Pinto beans	33
Butter beans	32 ± 3
Lentils	29 ± 3
Cashews	25 ± 1
Mixed nuts	24 ± 10
Kidney beans	22 ± 3

Beverages	Glycemic Index
Gatorade, orange flavor	89 ± 12
Rice milk	79 ± 8
Coca-Cola	63
Cranberry juice	59
Orange juice	50 ± 2
Soy milk	44 ± 5
Apple juice, unsweetened	41
Milk, full fat	41 ± 2
Skim milk	32
Tomato juice	31

Snack products	Glycemic Index
Tofu-based frozen dessert	115 ± 14

Pretzels	83 ± 9
Puffed rice cakes	82 ± 10
Jelly beans	80 ± 8
Licorice	78 ± 11
Pirate's Booty	70 ± 5
Angel food cake	67
Popcorn	65 ± 5
Water crackers	63 ± 9
Ice cream	62 ± 9
Potato chips	56 ± 3
Snickers bar	51
Milk chocolate, Dove	45 ± 8
Corn chips	42 ± 4
Low-fat yogurt	33 ± 3
M&M's peanut	33 ± 3
Dark chocolate, Dove	23 ± 3
Greek-style yogurt	12 ± 4
Hummus	6 ± 4

Meals	Glycemic Index
McDonald's hamburger	66 ± 8
Pizza Hut vegetarian supreme, thin and crispy	49 ± 6

GET SMART TO GET THINNER

"Limit sugar. Less bread. Less wine. More walking."

—Marcus

Choose high-fiber carbohydrates. High-fiber foods are one of your best weight-loss weapons. Years of research have found that the more fiber you eat, the better for your weight. How does dietary fiber fight fat?

First, it helps regulate the appetite hormone ghrelin, which tells you that you are hungry. Ghrelin levels are often out of whack in people with a high BMI so they always feel hungry no matter how much they eat. New research shows that high ghrelin levels not only make you feel hungrier, they also increase the desire for high-calorie foods compared with low-calorie fare, so it's a double whammy. But fiber can help. A 2009 study showed that eating a diet high in fiber helped balance ghrelin levels in overweight and obese people. This can turn off the constant hunger and reduce the appeal of high-calorie foods.

GET SMART TO GET THINNER

"I have been eating the Life-Enhancing Lentil Soup from your cookbook for lunch, and it keeps me feeling full. I don't get hungry two hours later like I used to."

—Fiona

Second, no matter how much you weigh, eating fiber helps you feel full longer so you don't get the munchies an hour after you eat.

Third, fiber slows the absorption of food into the bloodstream, which helps balance your blood sugar. This can help you make better food choices and fight cravings later in the day (see chapter 6 for more on this). In fact, fiber takes so long to be digested by your body, a person eating 20 to 35 grams of fiber a day will burn an extra 150 calories a day or lose 16 extra pounds a year.

These three things alone can go a long way in helping you avoid extra calories. Fiber-friendly foods boast a number of other health benefits as well, including:

- Reducing cholesterol
- Keeping your digestive tract moving
- Reducing high blood pressure
- Reducing the risk of cancer

Experts recommend eating 25–35 g of fiber a day, but research shows that most adults fall far short of that. So how can you boost your fiber intake? Eat more high-fiber brain healthy foods like fruits, vegetables, legumes, and whole grains. Here are the fiber contents of some brain healthy foods. Try to include some of the foods on this list at every meal or snack.

Food	Grams of Fiber
Kidney beans (1 cup canned)	16.4
Split peas (1 cup cooked)	16.4

Lentils (1 cup cooked)	15.6
Black beans (1 cup canned)	15.0
Garbanzo beans (1 cup canned)	10.6
Peas (1 cup frozen and cooked)	8.8
Raspberries (1 cup)	8.0
Blackberries (1 cup)	7.6
Spinach (1 cup cooked)	7.0
(1 cup raw)	0.7
Brussels sprouts (1 cup cooked)	6.4
Broccoli (1 cup cooked)	5.6
Pear (1 medium with skin)	5.1
Sweet potato (1 medium baked)	4.8
Carrots (1 cup cooked)	4.6
(1 medium raw)	2.0
Blueberries (1 cup)	3.5
Strawberries (1 cup)	3.3
Apple (1 medium with skin)	3.3
Banana (1 medium)	3.1
Orange (1 medium)	3.1
Asparagus (1 cup cooked)	3.0
Grapefruit (½ medium)	2.0
Avocado (1 ounce)	1.9
Whole wheat bread (1 slice)	1.9
Walnuts (7 whole)	1.9
Plums (2 medium)	1.8
Peach (1 medium with skin)	1.5
Tomato (½ cup fresh)	1.5
Cherries (10 large)	1.4
Oatmeal (¾ cup cooked)	0.8
Almonds (6 whole)	0.8

Source: *Adapted from U.S. Department of Agriculture, Agricultural Research Service,* USDA Nutritional Nutrient Database for Standard Reference, *Release 17, 2004.*

Steer clear of bad carbohydrates. Bad carbohydrates are those that have been robbed of any nutritional value, such as simple sugars and refined carbohydrates found in muffins, scones, cakes, cookies, and other baked goods. If you want to live without cravings, eliminate these completely from your diet.

Sugar is not your friend. We have often heard of sugar being called empty calories. In fact, it is so damaging to your brain and body that I call it anti-nutrition or toxic calories. Sugar increases inflammation in your body, increases erratic brain cell firing, and sends your blood sugar levels on a roller-coaster ride. Plus, new research shows that sugar is addictive and can even be *more* addictive than cocaine.

That helps explain why we eat so much of it. Americans consume an average of 22.2 teaspoons of sugar a day, which adds up to 355 calories a day. That's an increase of 19 percent since 1970.

NAMES FOR SUGAR USED ON FOOD LABELS

Invert sugar	Turbinado sugar
Lactose	Fructose
Maltodextrin	Agave
Honey	Dextrose
Maltose	Dehydrated cane juice
Glucose	Corn syrup
Malt syrup	High-fructose corn syrup
Galactose	Cane juice crystals, extract
Molasses	Cane sugar
Fruit juice concentrate	Sucanat
Sorbitol	Barley malt
Fruit juice	

Table sugar isn't the only culprit making you fat. Research shows that high-fructose corn syrup (HFCS), which is found in many sodas and accounts for as much as 40 percent of the caloric sweeteners used in the United States, is even more fattening than table sugar.

HFCS and sugar went head to head in a 2010 study from researchers at Princeton University. Compared with rats that drank water sweetened with table sugar, rats that drank water sweetened with HFCS gained significantly more body weight, including more fat around the belly, even though they consumed the same number of calories. Every single one of the rats drinking the HFCS became obese. After six months, the rats guzzling the HFCS showed signs of a dangerous condition known in humans as the metabolic syndrome, including weight gain, abdominal fat, and high triglycerides.

Put down the sodas and HFCS *now!*

A lot of people ask me, "Isn't it okay to have sweets in moderation?"

Personally, I don't agree with the people who say "Everything in moderation." Sugar in moderation triggers cravings. The less sugar in your life the better your life will be. Reach for a banana or an apple instead.

Cutting down on the sweet stuff is a good start, but sugar lurks in a lot of other processed foods as well like ketchup, barbecue sauce, and salad dressing. Start reading food labels. At first, you might feel like you're reading a foreign language. Sorbitol, maltose, maltidextrose, galactose—these are just some of the many names for sugar used on food labels.

RULE 5. FOCUS YOUR DIET ON HEALTHY FATS.

Healthy fats are important to a good diet because the solid weight of the brain is 60 percent fat! The one hundred billion nerve cells in your brain need essential fatty acids to function. Focus your diet on healthy fats, especially those that contain omega-3 fatty acids, found in foods like salmon, tuna, mackerel, avocados, walnuts, and green leafy vegetables.

How omega-3 fatty acids help you get thinner, smarter, and happier. The two most studied omega-3 fatty acids are eicosapentaenoic acid (EPA) and docosahexaenoic acid (DHA). DHA makes up a large portion of the gray matter of the brain. The fat in your brain forms cell membranes and plays a vital role in how our cells function. Neurons are also rich in omega-3 fatty acids. EPA improves blood flow, which boosts overall brain function.

Low levels of omega-3 fatty acids have been associated with depression, anxiety, obesity, ADD, suicide, and an increased risk for Alzheimer's disease and dementia. There is also scientific evidence that low levels of omega-3 fatty acids play a role in substance abuse, and I would argue that *overeating is a form of substance abuse.*

Boosting omega-3 fatty acids in your diet is one of the best things you can do for your weight, mood, and brainpower. In fact, if you want to lose fat, you should eat *more* fat—of the omega-3 variety. Increasing omega-3 intake has been found to decrease appetite and cravings and reduce body fat. In a fascinating 2009 study in the *British Journal of Nutrition,* Australian researchers analyzed blood samples from 124 adults (twenty-one healthy weight, forty overweight, and sixty-three obese), calculated their BMI, and measured their waist and hip circumference. They found that obese individuals had significantly lower levels of EPA and DHA compared with healthy-weight people. Subjects with higher levels were more likely to have a healthy BMI and waist and hip measurements.

GET SMART TO GET THINNER

"I never liked walnuts before. Now I love them!"

—Anna

Research in the last few years has revealed that diets rich in omega-3 fatty acids may help promote a healthy emotional balance and positive mood in later years, possibly because DHA is a main component of the brain's synapses. A growing body of scientific evidence indicates that fish oil helps ease symptoms of depression. One twenty-year study involving 3,317 men and women found that people with the highest consumption of EPA and DHA were less likely to have symptoms of depression.

There is a tremendous amount of scientific evidence pointing to a connection between the consumption of fish that is rich in omega-3 fatty acids and cognitive function. A Danish team of researchers compared the diets of 5,386 healthy older individuals and found that the more fish in a person's diet, the longer the person was able to maintain their memory and reduce the risk of dementia. Dr. J. A. Conquer and colleagues from the University of Guelph in Ontario, Canada, studied the blood fatty acid content in the early and later stages of dementia and noted low levels when compared with healthy people.

Eating fish also benefits cognitive performance. In a study from Swedish researchers, results showed that surveyed nearly five thousand fifteen-year-old boys and found that those who ate fish more than once a week scored higher on standard intelligence tests than teens who ate no fish. A follow-up study found that teens eating fish more than once a week also had better grades at school than students with lower fish consumption. Other benefits of omega-3 fatty acids include improving attention in people with ADD and reducing the risk for psychosis.

FOODS HIGH IN OMEGA-3 FATTY ACIDS

- Anchovies
- Broccoli
- Brussels sprouts
- Cabbage
- Cauliflower
- Cod
- Flaxseeds

- Halibut
- Mackerel
- Salmon, wild
- Sardines
- Scallops
- Shrimp
- Snapper
- Soybeans
- Spinach
- Tofu
- Trout
- Tuna
- Walnuts

Eat more fat, lose more fat. It sounds contradictory, but science shows that it's true. In 2000 researchers in Boston analyzed two groups of people—one group on a low-fat diet (20 percent of calories from fat) and the other group on a moderate-fat diet (35 percent of calories from fat). After eighteen months, people eating moderate amounts of fat lost a mean of 9 pounds and trimmed 2.7 inches from their waistlines. The low-fat group, however, *gained* a mean of 6.4 pounds and *added* 1 inch around the middle.

What I find intriguing about this study is that more than half of the moderate-fat dieters were able to stick with the program for the entire eighteen months. Compare that with 80 percent of the low-fat dieters who found it too hard to stick with the program and dropped out. I would venture to guess that the people eating moderate amounts of fat didn't feel like they were "dieting" because healthy fats help with satiety. The key to boosting fat consumption for weight loss is eating healthy fats.

Eliminate bad fats. While healthy fats enhance brainpower and help you lose weight, bad fats drain your brain and boost your belly. The U.S. Institute of Medicine recommends no more than 20 g saturated fat a day. Eating too many saturated fats or trans fats (also known as "Frankenfats") contributes to obesity and cognitive decline. Trans fats are used to help foods have a longer shelf life and are found in margarine, cakes, crackers, cookies, and potato chips. They decrease your shelf life!

Get rid of most animal fat from your diet. Diets high in saturated fats have long been associated with long-term health risks, such as heart disease. A recent animal study from British researchers has found that high-fat diets also cause more-immediate problems. After eating a fatty diet for just ten days, rats showed short-term memory loss and less energy to exercise—in other words, they became more stupid and lazy.

The researchers compared the performance of the rats on a high-fat diet (55 percent of calories as fat) with rats on a low-fat diet (7.5 percent of calories as fat). Rats with the high-fat diet had muscles that worked less efficiently, which lowered their energy levels, caused their hearts to work harder during exercise, and caused their hearts to increase in size. The rats eating high-fat foods also took longer to make their way through a maze and made more mistakes than the rats eating low-fat foods. This is one of the first studies to show that it doesn't take long for a high-fat diet to make your brain and body more sluggish.

GET SMART TO GET THINNER

"My secret to success has been reducing my intake of sugar, flour, bread, and red meat, and eating good fats, such as avocados and walnuts."

—Pete

Scientific evidence also shows that consuming high-fat foods actually alters brain chemistry in ways that compel you to overeat. One animal study that appeared in the *Journal of Clinical Investigation* found that eating high-fat foods, such as milkshakes or burgers, caused the brain to release messages to the body telling it to ignore the feelings of fullness that typically make you stop eating. In this particular study, the brain switched off the fullness signal for up to three days, which led to overeating.

A similar trial found that high-fat, high-sugar diets alter brain receptors in an area of the brain that regulates food intake. Overconsumption of fat-laden, sugar-filled foods increased the levels of opioid receptors, which are linked to feelings of pleasure and euphoria. The researchers suggest that this could be a factor in binge eating disorders.

What you eat doesn't just affect your own health. What you eat can affect your children . . . and their children. Research presented at the American Association for Cancer Research showed that the female offspring of pregnant rats that ate a diet high in omega-6 fats were more likely to get breast cancer. Omega-6 fats are found in vegetable oils, baked goods, and cereals. Even more disturbing is the finding that even if the daughters ate healthy diets, their female offspring were at a 30 percent higher risk for breast cancer.

This suggests that eating junk food could threaten not only your own health and well-being but that of your grandchildren. Other studies have shown that diets high in omega-6 compared with omega-3 fats raise the risk for depression and disease.

So after reading this, if you still want to grab that big Double-Double burger at In-N-Out, think about these facts:

- High-glycemic index of the white bun = 71
- Fat found in the 2 beef patties and 2 slices of cheese = 41 g
- Saturated fat = 18 g
- Trans fat = 1 g
- Calories = 670
- High-sodium content = 1,440 mg (milligrams)*

The daily limit of sodium should not exceed 1,500.

It makes you think twice about eating that burger, doesn't it? Knowledge is power. Know what you are putting in your mouth and how it will affect your brain and your belly.

GET SMART TO GET THINNER

"I started a vegetable garden at home and now I use the veggies in all kinds of things."

—Julie

RULE 6. EAT FROM THE RAINBOW.

This means put natural foods in your diet of many different colors. Eat blue foods (blueberries), red foods (pomegranates, strawberries, raspberries, cherries, red bell peppers, and tomatoes), yellow foods (squash, yellow bell peppers, bananas, and peaches), orange foods (oranges, tangerines, and yams), green foods (spinach, broccoli, and peas), purple foods (plums), and so on.

This will boost the antioxidant levels in your body and help keep your brain young. Several studies have found that eating foods rich in antioxidants, which include many fruits and vegetables, significantly reduces the risk of developing cognitive impairment.

Blueberries are very high in antioxidants, which has earned them the nickname "brain berries" among neuroscientists. In laboratory studies, rats that ate blueberries showed a better ability to learn new motor skills and gained protection against strokes. That is not all. In one study, rats that ate a diet rich in blueberries lost abdominal fat, lowered cholesterol, and improved glucose levels. Similar studies showed that rats that consumed strawberries and spinach also gained significant protection.

Eating fruits and vegetables from the rainbow, along with fish, legumes, and nuts is part of what is known as the Mediterranean diet. Research has found that eating a Mediterranean diet can make you not only happier but smarter too. A series of studies from Spanish researchers revealed that adherence to this type of eating plan helps prevent depression. A team of scientists in Bordeaux, France, concluded that a Mediterranean diet slows cognitive decline and reduces the risk for dementia.

FRUITS AND VEGETABLES WITH HIGH ANTIOXIDANT LEVELS

- Acai berries
- Avocados
- Beets
- Blueberries
- Blackberries
- Oranges
- Plums
- Pomegranates
- Raspberries
- Broccoli
- Brussels sprouts
- Cherries
- Cranberries
- Kiwis
- Red bell peppers
- Red grapes
- Strawberries
- Spinach

RULE 7. COOK WITH BRAIN HEALTHY HERBS AND SPICES TO BOOST YOUR BRAINPOWER.

If you want to get thinner, smarter, and happier, then reach for the spice cupboard. Using spices rather than heavy cream sauces or butter cuts calories so you can lose weight. Research shows that they can also boost your brain and your mood.

- **Turmeric** Found in curry, turmeric contains a chemical that has been shown to decrease the plaques in the brain thought to be responsible for Alzheimer's disease.
- **Saffron** In three studies, a saffron extract was found to be as effective as antidepressant medication in treating people with mild to moderate depression.

- **Sage** Scientific evidence shows that this fragrant spice helps to boost memory.

- **Thyme** Studies show that thyme increases the amount of DHA in the brain, which protects against age-related degeneration.

- **Rosemary** A 2006 study reported that rosemary diminishes cognitive decline in people with dementia.

- **Cinnamon** One of my favorite spices, cinnamon, has been shown to help boost attention. Plus, cinnamon is a natural aphrodisiac for men—not that most men need much help.

GET SMART TO GET THINNER

"Get creative with meal prep. I substitute healthier options for more traditional ingredients, like a vegetarian Reuben sandwich with raw zucchini, sprouts, and Vegenaise."

—Eddie

Other spices that boost or protect brainpower include garlic, oregano, and basil.

Brain Healthy Foods That Make You Thinner, Smarter, and Happier

Choosing brain healthy foods that will help you lose weight can also help you be smarter and happier. As you have noticed in this chapter, many of the foods mentioned have been found to improve cognitive function, reduce the risk of Alzheimer's disease and dementia, boost focus and attention, and more. There is no doubt in my mind that eating the right foods makes you smarter.

GET SMART TO GET THINNER

"I no longer buy foods that are bad for me. Period."

—Damon

In addition, you have probably noticed how the foods you eat affect your mood and energy level. That is because food is a drug. Food can make you feel worse. If you chow down on three doughnuts for breakfast, about half an hour later you are going to feel foggy, spacey, and stupid. Food can make you sleepy. Have you ever noticed that after wolfing down a huge lunch you feel like you need a nap? For some people, foods can trigger mood, temper control, attentional, or other emotional problems. This may be due to hidden food allergies or sensitivities.

In a 2008 study from Holland, researchers found that putting children on a restricted elimination diet reduced ADD symptoms by more than 50 percent in 73 percent of children—basically the same effectiveness of stimulant medication but without any of the side effects. The researchers also found that the children's moods and oppositional behaviors were also improved.

Elimination diets are not easy to do. For this study, the children could eat only rice, turkey, lamb, vegetables, fruits, margarine, vegetable oil, tea, pear juice, and water. But the results were stunning. An elimination diet may be a good place for you to start if you suspect food sensitivities. If you notice a reduction in your symptoms while on the elimination diet, then there is a good chance they are food-related. Adding foods back into your diet one by one will allow you to see which items may be causing the problem behaviors. Working with a nutritionist can make a big difference.

Food can also make you feel great. Eating brain healthy foods can lift your mood, improve focus and attention, and give you good energy that lasts all day long. For example, if you are feeling anxious or down in the dumps, sniff lemons. Research shows that the scent of lemons has antianxiety and antidepressant properties. In addition, foods that boost levels of the feel-good neurotransmitters serotonin and dopamine stabilize moods and rev up your energy. Healthy fare that pumps up the neurotransmitter GABA calms anxiety, which also makes you happier. For a real happiness boost, look for foods high in omega-3 fatty acids and vitamin B_{12}. Having low levels of omega-3s is associated with depression and obesity, and vitamin B_{12} deficiencies put you at higher risk for depression.

FIFTY BEST BRAIN HEALTHY FOODS

Almond milk, unsweetened	Lentils
Almonds, raw	Limes
Apples	Oats
Asparagus	Olive oil
Avocados	Oranges
Bananas	Peaches
Barley	Pears

Beans

Beets

Bell peppers

Blackberries

Blueberries

Bok choy

Broccoli

Brussels sprouts

Cherries

Chicken, skinless

Coconut

Coconut oil

Egg whites, DHA enriched

Goji berries

Grapefruit

Green tea

Herring

Kiwi

Lemons

Peas

Plums

Pomegranates

Quinoa

Raspberries

Red grapes

Salmon, wild

Soybeans

Spinach

Strawberries

Tomatoes

Tuna

Turkey, skinless

Walnuts

Water

Yams/sweet potatoes

Yogurt, low fat, sugar- and
    artificial-sweetener-free

GET SMART FOODS
(BRAIN HEALTHY FOODS THAT MAKE YOU
THINNER AND SMARTER)

Acai berries

Apples

Arugula

Avocados

Barley (pearled)

Beans

Beets

Blueberries

Blackberries

Broccoli

Brussels sprouts

Cauliflower

Cherries

Chicken (skinless)

Cinnamon

Cranberries

Eggs

Flaxseeds

Grape leaves

Green tea

Kiwis

Lean beef

Lentils

Mackerel

Milk (skim)

Oats

Oranges

Pecans

Pine nuts

Plums

Pomegranates

Raspberries

Red bell peppers

Red grapes

Rosemary

Saffron

Sage

Salmon

Sardines

Strawberries

Spinach

Thyme

Tomatoes

Tuna

Turkey (skinless)

Turmeric

Walnuts

Water

Whole grains

GOOD MOOD FOODS

(BRAIN HEALTHY FOODS THAT MAKE YOU THINNER AND HAPPIER)

Asparagus

Bananas

Beans

Broccoli

Cheese (low fat)

Chicken

Chickpeas

Cottage cheese (low fat)

Dark chocolate (not too much!)

Eggs

Lean meats

Lemons

Mackerel

Milk (skim)

Nuts

Oats

Protein

Pumpkin seeds

Saffron

Salmon

Sardines

Seafood

Spinach

Sunflower seeds

Tofu

Tuna

Using the lists in this chapter, create a list of your favorite brain healthy foods, good mood foods, and get smart foods. Use the chart below or a sheet of paper to write them down, or use the online nutrition tools on our website to find recipes with your top brain foods.

MY TOP 20 BRAIN FOODS

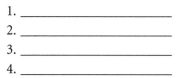

1. _____

2. _____

3. _____

4. _____

5. _____
6. _____
7. _____
8. _____
9. _____
10. _____
11. _____
12. _____
13. _____
14. _____
15. _____
16. _____
17. _____
18. _____
19. _____
20. _____

Brain Healthy Eating on a Budget

If you're concerned that buying brain healthy foods will bust your budget, stop worrying. You don't have to spend a bundle to eat right. I recently wrote a blog on brain healthy eating for the poor. In writing the blog, I asked for some help from my esteemed friend Dr. Jeff Fortuna, the author of *Nutrition for the Focused Brain* and *Food, Brain Chemistry and Behavior.* Dr. Fortuna is a faculty member in the Department of Health Science at California State University, Fullerton, and the clinical nutritionist for Newport Academy, a residential treatment program for teens suffering from drug abuse and co-occurring disorders. Together, we came up with the following ten tips to help people who are strapped for cash eat healthier without spending a fortune.

GO FOR SATISFYING GRAINS.

When it comes to grains, you can't beat old-fashioned oatmeal or pearled barley, which cost about ten cents or less per serving. These bargain whole grains offer a huge nutritional bang for your buck, moderate blood sugar for hours, and keep you feeling full longer.

BUY VITAMIN-RICH VEGETABLES FROZEN AND SAVE.

Stock up on frozen vegetables like broccoli, spinach, and carrots whenever you go to a warehouse store like Costco. It's cheaper than buying fresh and can cost you as little as eleven cents a serving.

BOOST ANTIOXIDANTS WITH APPLES, ORANGES, AND BANANAS.

Affordable apples and oranges (less than fifty cents each) and bananas (less than twenty cents each) are full of vitamins and antioxidants that promote health and boost brain performance.

SAY CHEESE—LOW-FAT COTTAGE CHEESE, THAT IS.

Cottage cheese is packed with protein, calcium, and vitamins A and D. With a single serving of cottage cheese, you get 13 g protein for about seventy-five cents. Just make sure you are one of the lucky ones who process dairy. Being lactose intolerant can drop blood flow to the brain and make you more impulsive.

PUMP UP PROTEIN WITH AFFORDABLE EGGS.

Getting adequate amounts of protein doesn't have to involve eating expensive meat. At less than twenty cents apiece, protein-rich eggs are an affordable option for breakfast, lunch, or dinner.

FILL UP ON HIGH-FIBER, LOW-COST BEANS.

Loaded with fiber and high in protein, beans should be a staple in any household that is struggling financially. For example, a 1-pound bag of black beans costs less than two dollars, and gives you twelve servings for less than sixteen cents each.

STOCK UP ON CANNED TUNA.

Eating fish like tuna is a great source of omega-3 fatty acids. You can get a three-pack of tuna for about $2.50, which means for about $.83 a can you get 22 grams of protein and a good amount of healthy omega-3 fatty acids. Be careful not to overdo the tuna as it may contain some mercury.

DRINK TO YOUR BRAIN HEALTH WITH SKIM MILK AND WATER.

Low in fat and high in protein and calcium, skim milk is fortified with vitamins A and D and will only set you back about twenty-five cents for one serving. You don't need to buy pricey bottled water. With a fifteen- to twenty-dollar water filter that fits on your kitchen faucet, you can drink from the tap and get healthy, filtered water that will keep your brain and body hydrated for optimal performance.

SPICE UP YOUR MEALS.

With just a few spices in your cupboard, you can enhance the flavor of any dish without using a lot of unhealthy butter, cream, or salt. You can find spices for a few dollars each—they're even cheaper if you can buy them loose where you scoop the spices into bags rather than buying them in a bottle.

BECOME A SAVVY SHOPPER.

You can save a bundle if you buy items that have a long shelf life—like canned tuna, beans, oatmeal, barley, and frozen vegetables—in bulk. Look for sales and specials, use coupons, and buy generic brands when possible. You can even shop online for many food items or look for coupons online from local stores to find the best deals.

Putting It All Together

Eating in a brain healthy way is about abundance, *not* deprivation. It is about great taste and wise spending. Your attitude here is critical. If you think of it as a loss of lasagna, you will not stick with it. But when you think of eating right as a *gain* in energy, a *gain* in happiness, and a *gain* in brainpower, you are much more likely to stay on track. The only thing you will lose is weight.

So how do you put this all together? Let me tell you what I do.

DR. AMEN'S TYPICAL BRAIN HEALTHY MEALS

- I have a protein powder and fruit shake for breakfast.
- I bring fresh-cut veggies with a little guacamole to work as a morning snack.
- I usually have a 350-calorie chicken, veggie, and avocado sandwich on nine-grain whole wheat bread with green tea for lunch.

- I have a piece of fruit and a few raw nuts as an afternoon snack.
- For dinner, I will often have a large salad or soup, plenty of veggies, and some form of protein like ahi tuna, wild salmon, or turkey if I need to focus in the evening. For the salad, I always put the dressing on the side. Why? I want to control the calories that go into my body.
- And I always have dessert—usually frozen blueberries with Greek yogurt.

GET SMART TO GET THINNER

"Track your calories in the *Daily Journal*. It really works!"

—Amy

With these brain healthy meals, I usually get eight or nine servings of fruits and veggies a day. It adds up to about 1,700 calories, which is slightly less than the 2,000 calories necessary to maintain my weight. Remember those rhesus monkeys? I want to be in the group with the better brain, so I choose to eat fewer calories. Plus, I have no cravings, which I truly love, and I feel happy and energetic.

To help you put it all together, here are my picks for the top fifteen brain healthy choices for breakfast, lunch, dinner, desserts, and snacks. You can find brain healthy recipes for some of the following in appendix E. Many of these delicious options come from *The Amen Solution Cookbook* or *Change Your Brain, Change Your Body Cookbook,* which include dozens of sumptuous recipes.

TOP FIFTEEN BRAIN HEALTHY CHOICES FOR BREAKFAST

- Daniel's Breakfast Shake (from *Change Your Brain, Change Your Body Cookbook;* see recipe in appendix E)
- Herb Garden Frittata with egg whites and veggies (from *Change Your Brain, Change Your Body Cookbook*)
- Dr. Amen's Low-Fat Southwestern Chicken Omelet (see recipe in appendix E)
- Almond Butter Quinoa (from *Change Your Brain, Change Your Body Cookbook;* see recipe in appendix E)

GET SMART TO GET THINNER

"When I started going online to look up the calories of the things I liked to order at my favorite restaurants, I was shocked. The turkey panini I liked was 900 calories! The tuna sandwich was 760 calories! That's too much! I found a nice Mediterranean salad at the same restaurant that has about 410 calories. If I hadn't looked it up, I never would have known how many extra calories I was eating."

—Shara

- Feed Your Brain Breakfast Burrito with egg whites, veggies, avocado, and whole-grain tortillas (from *Change Your Brain, Change Your Body Cookbook*)
- Steel-cut oatmeal with walnuts, blueberries, and unsweetened almond milk
- Feel-Good Eggs Ranchero (from *The Amen Solution Cookbook*; see recipe in appendix E)
- Barley cooked with apples, dried cranberries, pecans, cinnamon, and unsweetened almond milk
- Egg whites, turkey bacon, and whole wheat toast
- Egg whites, black beans, fresh salsa, and avocado
- Unsweetened Greek yogurt, berries, and chopped almonds
- Low-fat cottage cheese and fruit
- Red, White, and Blue Smoothie (see recipe in appendix E)
- Almond butter and banana sandwich on whole wheat
- Brain Berry Decadence (see recipe in appendix E)

TOP FIFTEEN BRAIN HEALTHY CHOICES FOR LUNCH

- Smart Spinach Salad (from *Change Your Brain, Change Your Body Cookbook*; see recipe in appendix E)
- Turkey sandwich on whole wheat with mustard, spinach, tomatoes, and avocado
- Brain Fitness Fajita Salad (from *The Amen Solution Cookbook*; see recipe in appendix E)

- Quick Wit Quinoa Salad with black beans, cherry tomatoes, pine nuts, avocado, red bell pepper, celery, green onion, and lime juice vinaigrette (from *Change Your Brain, Change Your Body Cookbook*)

- Magnificent Mind Cucumber Mint Salad (from *Change Your Brain, Change Your Body Cookbook;* see recipe in appendix E)

- Scrumptious Southwestern Tacos with lettuce "shells," chicken breast, tomatoes, low-fat cheese, fresh salsa, and avocado (from *Change Your Brain, Change Your Body Cookbook*)

- Chicken breast sandwich on whole wheat pita bread with hummus, cucumber, and olives

- Turkey burger with ground white meat turkey on multigrain bun with mustard, lettuce, tomato, and low-fat cheese

- Mindful Minestrone Soup (from *The Amen Solution Cookbook;* see recipe in appendix E)

- Life-Enhancing Lentil Soup with celery, red bell pepper, onions, brown rice, and spices (from *Change Your Brain, Change Your Body Cookbook*)

- Albacore tuna wrap sandwich on whole wheat tortilla with Vegenaise, celery, apples, and dried cranberries

- Very Veggie Sandwich (see recipe in appendix E)

- Chicken breast fajitas on whole wheat tortilla with bell peppers, onions, salsa, and avocado

- Tofu stir-fry with broccoli and mushrooms

- Hard-boiled egg white sandwich on toasted whole wheat bread with Vegenaise, celery, and green onions

TOP FIFTEEN BRAIN HEALTHY CHOICES FOR DINNER

- Tana's Smooth Sweet Potato Soup (from *Change Your Brain, Change Your Body Cookbook,* see recipe in appendix E)

- Ginger Glazed Salmon with ginger root, lemon juice, Dijon mustard, soy sauce, and honey—serve with quinoa and sautéed spinach (from *Change Your Brain, Change Your Body Cookbook*)

- Smart Brain Spaghetti with spaghetti squash (spaghetti squash looks like pasta but has more nutrients), red bell peppers, zucchini, onion, tomatoes, tomato sauce, and spices—add grilled turkey breast or chicken breast for protein boost (from *Change Your Brain, Change Your Body Cookbook*)

- Poached Tilapia in Saffron Sauce with tomatoes, fennel, leek, okra, and lemon—serve with steamed broccoli and barley (from *Change Your Brain, Change Your Body Cookbook*)
- Get Smart Mahi Mahi Burger with Pineapple Salsa (from *The Amen Solution Cookbook;* see recipe in appendix E)
- Healthy Turkey Chili (from *Change Your Brain, Change Your Body Cookbook;* see recipe in appendix E)
- Stuffed Vegetables with bell peppers, zucchini, Japanese eggplant, and crookneck squash filled with a lean ground lamb, barley, and spices mixture (from *Change Your Brain, Change Your Body Cookbook*)
- JT's Grilled Salmon (see recipe in appendix E)
- Chili Lime Chicken with Veggie Kabobs with chicken breast, bell peppers, zucchini, squash, mushrooms, and onions (from *Change Your Brain, Change Your Body Cookbook*)
- Savory Lubian Rose Lamb Stew (from *The Amen Solution Cookbook;* see recipe in appendix E)
- Seared Ahi with Guacamole—serve with steamed asparagus (from *Change Your Brain, Change Your Body Cookbook*)
- Coconut Curry Noodles with spaghetti squash, broccoli, carrots, asparagus, red bell peppers, squash, bok choy, and snow peas in a ginger, soy, coconut sauce (from *Change Your Brain, Change Your Body Cookbook*)
- Turkey Meatloaf with lean ground turkey, oats, onion, eggs, spices, and a tomato sauce—serve with a side salad (from *Change Your Brain, Change Your Body Cookbook*)
- Salmon Curry Chowder with carrots, onion, celery, potatoes, peas, and spinach in a coconut curry broth (from *Change Your Brain, Change Your Body Cookbook*)
- Grilled tofu in a soy ginger sauce (serve with shiitake mushrooms and broccoli)

TOP FIFTEEN BRAIN HEALTHY SNACKS

- Chopped veggies and hummus
- Soaked raw almonds

- Fresh guacamole and red bell peppers
- Celery with almond butter
- Apple slices or a banana with almond butter
- Unsweetened yogurt and blueberries
- Deviled eggs with hummus (discard the yolk)
- Turkey and apple slices with a few almonds
- Cottage cheese and fruit
- Protein shake
- Baked sweet potato chips with fresh salsa
- Steamed edamame
- Fresh guacamole on sprouted grain toast
- Homemade turkey jerky
- Meal-replacement protein bar with low sugar content

GET SMART TO GET THINNER

"The *Daily Journal* is like having someone with you on a daily basis to say you did that right or you could do better there."

—Yuko

TOP FIFTEEN BRAIN HEALTHY DESSERTS

- Scintillating Sugar-Free Sorbet (from *Change Your Brain, Change Your Body Cookbook;* see recipe in appendix E)

- Banana Ice Dream Sundae with frozen bananas, dates, almonds, and fruit—blend and freeze like Popsicles! (from *Change Your Brain, Change Your Body Cookbook*)

- Chocolate Nut Ice Dream Bars with frozen bananas, almond butter, carob powder, yogurt, chocolate almond milk, and chocolate stevia—blend and freeze like Popsicles! (from *Change Your Brain, Change Your Body Cookbook*)

- EZ Blueberry Ice Cream (from *Change Your Brain, Change Your Body Cookbook;* see recipe in appendix E)

- Low-fat cottage cheese with peach slices

- Choco-Berry Brain-Biotic Shake with chocolate almond milk, coconut milk ice cream, protein powder, and fruit (from *Change Your Brain, Change Your Body Cookbook*)

- Banana and almond butter

- Unsweetened yogurt with fresh berries and chopped almonds

- Low-sugar dark chocolate (only a small amount!)

- Apple slices and low-fat cheese

- Berries served warm with muesli made from oats, almonds, and sunflower seeds with a touch of honey

- Tana's Green Chai Latte with almond milk and flavored stevia (from *Change Your Brain, Change Your Body Cookbook*)

- Chocolate-Covered Strawberry Mousse with tofu, almond milk, carob powder, almond butter, and stevia (from *Change Your Brain, Change Your Body Cookbook*)

- Snappy Coconut Strawberry Smoothie with yogurt, strawberries, coconut milk, and coconut flakes (from *Change Your Brain, Change Your Body Cookbook*)

- Fresh fruit salad

GET SMART TO GET THINNER

"If I'm ever wondering why I gained a few pounds I can just go back to my *Daily Journal* and see that, for example, when I skipped my workout two days in a row and ate this particular food, well, that's how I gained those extra pounds."

—Sherisse

Journaling: A Critical Part of the Amen Solution

Keeping a food journal helps you avoid calorie amnesia. You know, the handful of nuts you grabbed from the receptionist's desk, the 200-calorie sports drink you downed after your workout, the glass of wine you drank while preparing dinner. Since they weren't part of your "meals," you may not remember that you consumed these calories. Then when you aren't losing weight, you wonder why. "I only ate a total of 1,800 calories for breakfast, lunch, and dinner. What's the problem?" The problem is calorie amnesia. Keeping a food diary is the answer.

Tracking your calories in a food journal also *doubles* your weight loss, according to a 2008 study from Kaiser Permanente's Center for Health Research. Writing down everything that goes into your body for ten weeks makes you conscious, aware, and more likely to do the right things. It holds you accountable.

A food journal also helps you track your progress. You can flip through it and see how much better you are doing—how many brain healthy fruits and vegetables you are eating, how you have replaced trans fats with healthy fats, how you have lowered your overall calorie intake. Seeing your progress is a tremendous motivator that will keep you going in the right direction.

GET SMART TO GET THINNER

"In the *Daily Journal* there's a list of 'weight boosters.' I had almost everything on that list—low thyroid, low blood sugar, imbalanced hormones, trouble sleeping, negative thinking. No wonder I wasn't losing weight before."

—Carrie

The compelling evidence about the effectiveness of keeping a food diary is part of what inspired me to create *The Amen Solution Daily Journal.* It helps you keep track of your calories, and a *lot* more. After working with thousands of patients, I have discovered that tracking not just your calories, but also your physical activity, energy levels, sleep, and ANTs can help keep you motivated and improve your success. I have also found that daily reminders significantly increase the likelihood that you will follow through with your new brain healthy habits.

For example, in our *Daily Journal,* there is a checklist with reminders about what you need to do on a daily basis to improve your brain health. This list includes:

- Review your One-Page Miracle so you can stay focused on what is important to you
- Take your brain healthy supplements, including a multivitamin and fish oil
- Do a daily meditation to calm your mind and increase your focus
- Drink your daily water requirement, which is half your weight in ounces

The journal I created is designed to make you more successful in your efforts to lose weight, be happier, and boost your brain. It should take no more than five minutes to complete the daily entry and will give you a complete snapshot of your journey to better brain health and a better body. At the end of this chapter are sample pages from *The Amen Solution Daily Journal* to help get you started.

GET SMART TO GET THINNER

"I interacted with my *Daily Journal*. If it said to take a multivitamin, I wrote 'okie-dokie' next to that. If it said to eat healthy fats like avocado, I wrote 'yummy' in the margin. It was an interactive experience for me."

—Colleen

Many of our weight-loss participants say the journal is the most important tool in our entire program. Sharon is one of them, and she says the time it requires to fill out each day is well worth the effort. She says that if the number on her scale starts going in the wrong direction, she can review her journal, figure out where she went wrong, and get back on track. So many people think they are doing the right things and don't understand why the number on the scale is creeping up, but when you write down your daily behaviors and food intake, it often becomes glaringly clear where you can make improvements.

Sharon also found that recording her daily energy levels in the journal helped her identify a regularly occurring energy lull in the afternoons. She says she never would have noticed it if she hadn't been keeping track. She brought up the issue in our weight-loss group, made a few recommended tweaks to her program, and boosted her afternoon energy level.

Log on for long-term weight loss. Keeping a daily journal online can be just as helpful as using a pen-and-paper variety. In 2010 the researchers at Kaiser Permanente found that patients who logged on to an online weight-loss support group and tracked their efforts maintained the greatest weight loss. It was findings like these that inspired me to create interactive tools on our website so you can fill out the *Daily Journal* online to keep track of your progress. The site also offers calorie counters, brain healthy meal planners, and much more to support you in your efforts.

So whether you are more comfortable with a pen-and-paper journal you can tote with you in your briefcase or handbag, or an online interactive tracking program, the bottom line is, use it every day for greater weight loss.

The Amen Solution All-Stars: Rhona

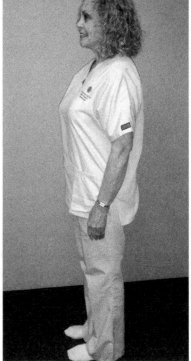

| Start, 141 pounds | After two ten-week cycles, lost 9 pounds |

Sixty-seven-year-old Rhona didn't have much weight to lose when she joined our weight loss group. At 5'1" and 141 pounds, her BMI was 27, which put her in the overweight category but not far off from a healthy BMI. Rhona had spent a lifetime losing weight and gaining it back. When she was younger, she could drop 10 pounds in a couple of weeks, but as she got older, it got harder to shed the extra baggage. She was hoping the Amen Solution would be the answer.

Rhona's answers on the questionnaire didn't reveal a specific brain type, so she followed a general brain healthy program that included the Amen Clinics Seven Rules for Brain Healthy Eating, exercising for thirty minutes five to six times a week, taking fish oil and vitamin D, and using the *Daily Journal*.

For Rhona, journaling proved to be the secret to success. "The best part of the program was the journal," she said. "The journal is the most important tool. That book is so thorough. I got so into it and never missed one day. It kept me aware, motivated, inspired, and on track. I would write what I was feeling, what sabotaged me yesterday, and how I was going to fix it tomorrow. There are a million journals out there but none of them are even close to being as thorough as this one. It isn't just a tool for the program; it's a lifetime tool."

With the help of the *Daily Journal,* Rhona lost 5 pounds after ten weeks and dropped another 4 pounds over the following ten weeks for a total weight loss of 9 pounds. But the weight loss isn't the only thing she gained from the program.

"I never expected to learn so much. After learning about how to feed my brain, I will never be the same," she said. "Now I think twice before I put anything in my mouth and ask myself, 'Does this feed my brain or dehydrate it?'" Some of her favorite brain healthy foods? Blueberries, red and orange bell peppers, and nuts—things she never had in her kitchen before.

Going through the program has also boosted her happiness quotient. Writing in the journal (which includes a daily gratitude exercise) every morning gets her day off on the right foot. "Now when I wake up, it is in gratitude. That's how I start my day. I celebrate my successes and celebrate what I am eating because I know it is good for my brain."

SAMPLE PAGES FROM
THE AMEN SOLUTION DAILY JOURNAL

DATE:

Time	Food & Beverages	Calories	Healthy? (Yes/No)
	Breakfast		
	Snack		
	Lunch		
	Snack		
	Dinner		
	Other		
Calories Allowed:		Today's Calories:	

My Brain Healthy Reminders

Tip of the day: Love Your Brain

Today's Weight: _____   Hours Slept Last Night: _____

- ☐ Review One-Page Miracle
- ☐ Take brain healthy supplements
- ☐ Stay within calorie budget
- ☐ Drink water requirement

- ☐ Kill the ANTs
- ☐ Do daily meditation
- ☐ Eat brain healthy foods
- ☐ Learn something new
- ☐ Get 30 minutes of exercise

WORKOUT

Physical Activity	Minutes	Calories Burned

WRITE 5 THINGS THAT I AM GRATEFUL FOR TODAY:

1. _____
2. _____
3. _____
4. _____
5. _____

WRITE 1 THING THAT MOTIVATES ME TODAY:

_____

On a scale of 1–10 (1 is terrible, 10 is great) rate your:

Quality of Sleep	1	2	3	4	5	6	7	8	9	10
Mood	1	2	3	4	5	6	7	8	9	10
Anxiety	1	2	3	4	5	6	7	8	9	10
Attention	1	2	3	4	5	6	7	8	9	10
Energy	1	2	3	4	5	6	7	8	9	10
Memory	1	2	3	4	5	6	7	8	9	10
Self-Control	1	2	3	4	5	6	7	8	9	10

4

KNOW YOUR BRAIN TYPE

ONE SIZE DOES *NOT* FIT EVERYONE

When I first started to do our brain imaging work at the Amen Clinics in 1991 I was looking for the one pattern that was associated with depression, ADD, or bipolar disorder. But as I soon discovered there was clearly not one brain pattern associated with any of these illnesses. They all had multiple types.

As we looked at the brains of our overweight patients, we again discovered that again there was not one brain pattern associated with being overweight; there were at least five different types. We saw patterns associated with brains that tended to be compulsive, some that were impulsive, some that were sad, and others that were anxious—in various combinations.

This is exactly the reason why most diets don't work. They take a one-size-fits-all approach, which from our brain imaging work makes absolutely no sense at all.

A Radical New Look

Have you ever gone on a diet with a friend only to see her successfully drop pound after pound while you struggle to lose a single ounce? And she feels energized and focused while you end up feeling irritated and emotional all the time? You probably beat yourself up about it, thinking you were doing something wrong or weren't trying hard enough, even though you did exactly what was recommended. Your diet buddy might have even accused you of cheating to explain why you didn't lose any weight. After all, the diet plan was working for her, so why shouldn't it work for you?

I can explain why it might have worked for your friend but not for you. The whole notion that one weight-loss program, diet plan, treatment, or method can work for everyone is ridiculous. Giving everyone the same diet plan will make some people better, but it will also make a lot of people worse. So the diet you and your friend tried was probably right for her brain but wrong for your brain.

GET SMART TO GET THINNER

"I read your book and started making some of the changes suggested for the 'problems' that I have related to my brain. I have introduced what I have learned so far, and I have lost 7 pounds in the last ten days. I feel so much better! I would like to lose another 15–18 pounds. This would put me at the lower end of normal for my BMI—a place I have not been in many years."

—Claudia

Other scientists are finally beginning to wake up to the radical idea that weight-loss plans need to be individualized. A 2010 study on fruit flies appearing in the journal *Genetics* reported that rather than diet alone, it was the way genes interacted with various diets that had the greatest influence on body weight. Another team of researchers from Stanford University found that some people have a genetic predisposition to respond better to a low-carb diet while others benefit more from a low-fat diet. In this 2010 trial involving 133 overweight women, women who ate a diet that matched their genetic predisposition lost 5.3 percent of their body weight compared with 2.3 percent for women eating a diet that conflicted with their genetic predisposition. These two studies back up the concept that when it comes to weight loss, one size does *not* fit all.

Knowing about your own specific brain is the key to losing weight and keeping it off. It can make it so much easier for you to follow a healthy eating plan. In this chapter you will learn about each of the five types of overeaters, including types of diets that could be sabotaging your weight-loss efforts and eating plans that that will help you shed the pounds. In addition, I will introduce you to behavioral interventions, natural supplements, and when necessary, medications targeted for each brain type to help you stay on track.

Before I describe the five types, I'm going to give you a crash course in Brain 101 so you can understand the brain systems that play a major role in

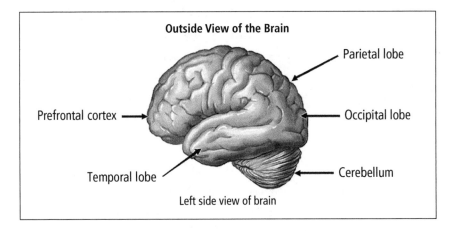

Outside View of the Brain

Parietal lobe

Prefrontal cortex

Occipital lobe

Temporal lobe

Cerebellum

Left side view of brain

your behavior. All of these systems can either help or hurt your ability to lose weight and keep it off.

PREFRONTAL CORTEX (PFC)

Think of the PFC as the CEO of your brain. Situated at the front third of your brain, it supervises your life. It is involved with forethought, judgment, impulse control, planning, attention, follow-through, organization, empathy, and learning from the mistakes you make. The PFC is like the brain's brakes. It stops us from saying stupid things or making bad decisions. It is the little voice in your head that helps you decide between the peach and the peach cobbler.

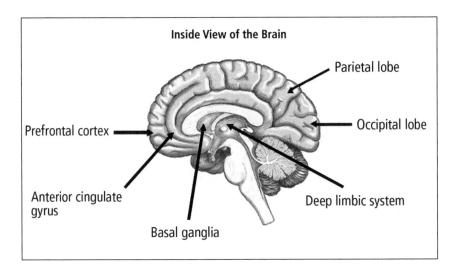

Inside View of the Brain

Parietal lobe

Prefrontal cortex

Occipital lobe

Anterior cingulate gyrus

Basal ganglia

Deep limbic system

When the PFC works well, it helps you say no to double cheeseburgers and chocolate pie. When there is low activity in the PFC, it is linked to a lack of clear goals, procrastination, a short attention span, bad judgment, impulsivity, and not learning from the mistakes you make, which makes you more likely to engage in habits that make you overweight, unhappier, and less intelligent. Alcohol lowers activity in the PFC, which is why people do such stupid things when they get drunk.

One of my patients with bulimia tells me that when she goes out to drink with her friends, she often eats more than she wants and subsequently makes herself throw up when she gets home. Avoid those things that lower PFC function (alcohol, lack of sleep, brain injuries, etc.).

ANTERIOR CINGULATE GYRUS (ACG)

I call the ACG the brain's gear shifter. It runs lengthwise through the deep parts of the frontal lobes and allows us to shift our attention and be flexible and adaptable and to change when needed. When there is too much activity in this part of the brain, people tend to become stuck on negative thoughts or negative behaviors, they tend to worry, hold grudges, and be oppositional or argumentative. It also may make them more vulnerable to being obsessive or struggle with compulsive behaviors, and it has been linked to eating disorders, such as anorexia. The ACG is also involved in error detection and lets you know when something is wrong or out of place. If it works too hard you tend to see too many problems. For example, when some women are premenstrual, serotonin levels go low, which increases ACG activity and makes them overfocused on what makes them unhappy.

One of my friends has a very active ACG. She sees way too many errors in her husband and children. Until we are able to calm this part of her brain, nothing will help her be happy.

DEEP LIMBIC SYSTEM

Lying near the center of the brain, the deep limbic system is involved in setting a person's emotional tone. When this area is less active, people tend to be more positive and hopeful. When it is overactive, negativity can take over and lower motivation and drive, decrease self-esteem, and increase feelings of guilt and helplessness. Abnormalities in the limbic brain have been associated with mood disorders.

BASAL GANGLIA

Surrounding the deep limbic system, the basal ganglia are involved with integrating thoughts, feelings, and movements. This part of the brain is also involved in setting a person's anxiety level. When there is too much activity in the basal ganglia, people tend to struggle with anxiety and physical stress symptoms, such as headaches, stomachaches, and muscle tension. High anxiety often sets the stage for overeating, especially sugary, high-carbohydrate foods that have a calming effect. People may overeat to settle their fears or to relieve tension. This area is also involved with feelings of pleasure and ecstasy.

Cocaine works in this part of the brain to release the pleasure chemical dopamine. Cookies, cakes, and other sugar-laden, fat-filled treats also activate this area. Some trials suggest that sugar is actually *more* addictive than cocaine. For example, a 2007 study conducted by a team of French researchers found that when rats were allowed to choose between cocaine and water sweetened with either saccharin or sucrose, the vast majority of them (94 percent) chose the sweetened beverages over the cocaine. Not even increases in the doses of cocaine could lure the rats away from the sweet stuff.

TEMPORAL LOBES

The temporal lobes, located underneath your temples and behind your eyes, are involved with language, short-term memory, mood stability, and temper issues. They are part of the brain's "what pathway," because they help you recognize and name "what" things are. Normal activity in this area generally results in stable moods and an even keel. Trouble in the temporal lobes often leads to memory problems, mood instability, and temper problems.

PARIETAL LOBES

The parietal lobes toward the top back part of the brain are involved with sensory processing and direction sense. They are called the "where pathway" in the brain, because they help you know where things are in space, such as navigating your way to the kitchen at night in the dark. The parietal lobes are one of the first areas damaged by Alzheimer's disease, which is why people with this condition tend to get lost. They have also been implicated in eating disorders and self-body distortion syndromes, such as with anorexics who think they are fat.

OCCIPITAL LOBES

Located at the back of the brain, the occipital lobes are involved with vision and visual processing.

CEREBELLUM

Located at the back bottom part of the brain, the cerebellum is involved with physical coordination, thought coordination, and processing speed. There are large connections between the PFC and the cerebellum, which is why many scientists think that the cerebellum is also associated with judgment and impulse control. When there are problems in the cerebellum, people tend to struggle with physical coordination, slow processing, and have trouble learning. Alcohol is directly toxic to this part of the brain, which is why drunk people usually fail sobriety tests that involve balance and coordination moves like balancing on one leg or touching their fingertip to their nose. Improving the cerebellum through coordination exercises can improve your prefrontal cortex and also help your judgment and your body.

BRIEF BRAIN SYSTEM SUMMARY

- Prefrontal cortex—judgment, forethought, planning, and impulse control
- Anterior cingulate gyrus—shifting attention and error detection
- Deep limbic system—sets emotional tone, involved with mood and bonding
- Basal ganglia—integrates thoughts, feelings, and movements, involved with pleasure
- Temporal lobes—memory, mood stability, and temper issues, "what pathway"
- Parietal lobes—sensory processing and direction sense, "where pathway"
- Occipital lobes—vision and visual processing
- Cerebellum—motor coordination, thought coordination, processing speed, and judgment

Summary of the Amen Clinics Five Types of Overeaters

Take the questionnaire in appendix A to see if you fit into a specific type or if you have more than one type, which is common. Based on your answers, you will be better able to tailor this program for your individual needs so you can finally get thinner, smarter, and happier.

Type 1. Compulsive Overeaters

People with this type tend to get stuck on thoughts of food. They hear the ice cream in the freezer calling their name—over and over and over again. They get so focused on the French fries they are going to order for lunch that they forget to join their 11 a.m. conference call. They often feel compulsively driven to eat and often say they have no control over food. They also tend to be nighttime eaters because they worry and have trouble sleeping.

GET SMART TO GET THINNER

"No matter what, I just couldn't stop thinking about food."

—Hannah

The basic mechanism of this type is that they tend to get stuck on thoughts or locked into one course of action. In addition to getting stuck on thoughts about food, they may also get stuck on their worries. They tend to be rigid, inflexible, have trouble seeing options, and feel like they *must* have things their way, or they get upset.

This type is also associated with holding grudges and having problems with oppositional or argumentative behavior. This means that no matter what you ask them, their first response is almost always automatically no. Even if you ask them something that you know they will like, such as if they want to go to their favorite restaurant for dinner, they will probably say no.

BRAIN SPECT FINDINGS FOR COMPULSIVE OVEREATERS

SPECT scans show that compulsive overeaters generally have too much activity in the front part of their brains, especially in the ACG. When there is too much activity in this area, people tend to become stuck on negative thoughts or actions. Overactivity in this part of the brain is most commonly caused by low levels of the neurotransmitter serotonin.

Healthy Scan

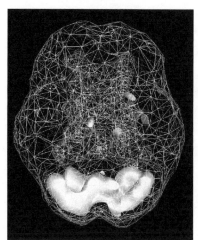

Good activity in the cerebellum,
cool everywhere else

Compulsive Overeater

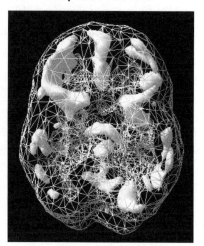

Increased anterior cingulate gyrus
and prefrontal activity

This view is called our active scan, looking at areas of increased activity. Gray indicates average activity, whereas white indicates the top 15 percent. In this view we are looking up from the bottom, where the top is the front part of the brain and the bottom is the back part of the brain. In a healthy scan in adults, the back part of the brain (cerebellum) is usually the most active. In compulsive overeaters generally there is too much activity in the front part of their brains so they have trouble overthinking.

WHAT MAKES COMPULSIVE OVEREATERS WORSE

The following types of diets, beverages, supplements, and medications can make this type worse and make it almost impossible to stick to a weight-loss plan.

- High-protein diets, which tend to be concentration diets and help people focus. On diets like the Atkins diet, compulsive overeaters focus more on the things that upset them. This doesn't mean you should avoid protein completely, just focus more on healthy carbohydrates. I was on *The Rachael Ray Show* in 2010 talking about different brain types. When I mentioned that certain diets can make people worse, Rachael became very animated and said, "I tried that no-carb, low-carb diet for three days and I was the most angry, irritable person. I am lucky my husband didn't leave me."

- Caffeinated beverages or caffeine pills
- Diet pills, such as phentermine
- Stimulants, such as Ritalin or Adderall

WHAT WORKS FOR COMPULSIVE OVEREATERS

Compulsive overeaters do best when we find natural ways to increase serotonin, which is calming to the brain. In addition, learning how to get unstuck from thoughts about food and worries can be helpful.

- Eat complex carbohydrates and other brain healthy foods that help the body produce more serotonin, such as these recommended by my friend and colleague Dr. Eric Braverman, author of *Younger You:*

    - Bananas
    - Beets
    - Brown rice
    - Cottage cheese (I recommend 1% or fat-free)
    - Herbal teas
    - Mackerel
    - Salmon
    - Sunflower seeds
    - Swiss cheese (I recommend low fat)
    - Turkey (I recommend skinless)

- Get enough physical exercise, which boosts serotonin levels. (See chapter 7 for more on which types of exercise are best for this type.)
- Avoiding nighttime eating after dinner. New research suggests that people who eat late at night gain even more weight than people who eat the same number of calories during the day. It seems that eating late at night throws off your internal clock so that your body decides to store more fat. I know many people who say that the only time they feel hungry is at night, but that is usually because they have a lot of bad brain habits, like skipping breakfast or going too long in between meals.
- If you get a thought in your head more than three times, do something to distract yourself.
- Make a list of ten things you can do instead of eating so you can distract yourself.

- People with this type always do better with choices, rather than edicts. Do not tell them where you are going to eat or what they are going to eat; give them choices.

- Avoid automatically opposing others or saying no, even to yourself.

- If you have trouble sleeping, try a glass of warm milk with a teaspoon of vanilla and a few drops of stevia.

- Supplements, such as 5-HTP, the B vitamin inositol, and saffron, L-tryptophan, and St. John's wort increase serotonin. In fact, there is good scientific evidence that indicates 5-HTP helps with weight loss, and in my experience, I have found that it works best for this type. (See chapter 5 for more on how these supplements work.)

- When other interventions do not work, serotonin-enhancing medications, such as Prozac, Zoloft, Celexa, or Lexapro can be helpful.

MEET AMY, A COMPULSIVE OVEREATER

Amy is an ICU nurse who fit this type perfectly. She felt as though she couldn't stop herself from eating and thought about food constantly throughout the day. She likened her thoughts to a little mouse on an exercise wheel; even though the mouse was exhausted, he couldn't get off. Caffeine and diet pills made Amy anxious because her brain did not need more stimulation. She often felt as though she needed a glass of wine at night—or two or three—to calm her worries. No diet would work for Amy long term until we calmed her brain. Using the strategies listed above, Amy lost 45 pounds over a year.

GET SMART TO GET THINNER

"If I saw food, I ate it. Now I can look at it and say no."

—John

Type 2. Impulsive Overeaters

People with this type struggle with impulsivity and have trouble controlling their behavior, even though they begin each day with good intentions to eat well. People with this type don't think about food constantly, but whenever they see it, they can't resist. If they drive past their favorite burger joint, they are likely to stop even if they aren't really hungry. They have a hard time saying no when someone offers them a second—or third or fourth—slice of pizza, piece of cake, or helping of mashed potatoes.

One of my best friends is a perfect example of this type. He is on a diet every single day of his life. He wakes up every morning committed to the idea of eating right. He maintains that thought as he passes the first doughnut shop, but then he starts to sweat as he passes the second doughnut shop, and by the time he passes the third one he has no willpower left. After completely giving up on his plans by noon, he utters the famous words of all impulsive overeaters: "I'll start my diet . . . tomorrow."

SPECT FINDINGS FOR IMPULSIVE OVEREATERS

The most common brain SPECT finding in this type is decreased activity in the PFC, which is most commonly associated with low levels of the neurotransmitter dopamine. Impulsive overeating is common among people who have ADD, which has also been associated with low dopamine levels in the brain. People with ADD struggle with a short attention span, distractibility, disorganization, and impulsivity.

Research suggests that having untreated ADD nearly doubles the risk for being overweight. Without proper treatment, it is nearly impossible for these people to be consistent with any nutrition plan. My research team and I have published several studies showing that when people with ADD try to concentrate they actually get less activity in the PFC, which will cause them to have even less control over their own behavior. For these people, literally, the harder they try to lose weight the worse it gets.

Impulsive overeaters may also be the result of some form of toxic exposure, a near-drowning accident, a brain injury to the front part of the brain, or a brain infection, such as chronic fatigue syndrome. Overweight smokers and heavy coffee drinkers also tend to fit this type.

WHAT MAKES IMPULSIVE OVEREATERS WORSE

Anything that boosts serotonin in the brain will calm the brain and make this type worse because it can lower both your worries and your impulse control, giving new meaning to the term *fat and happy*. Things that deplete dopamine levels are also a problem. These include:

- High-carbohydrate diets
- Alcohol, caffeine, and sugar deplete dopamine

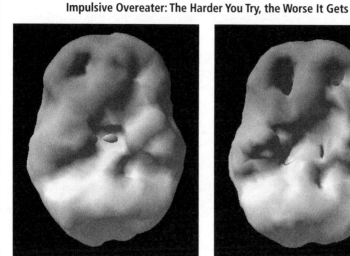

Impulsive Overeater: The Harder You Try, the Worse It Gets

At rest   With concentration

Notice that with concentration there is overall decreased activity, especially in the prefrontal cortex at the top of the image.

- Stress
- Serotonin-enhancing supplements, such as 5-HTP
- Serotonin-enhancing medications, such as Prozac, Zoloft, or Lexapro

WHAT WORKS FOR IMPULSIVE OVEREATERS

We help impulsive overeaters by boosting dopamine levels and strengthening the prefrontal cortex.

- Eat brain healthy foods that are high in phenylalanine and tyrosine, the building blocks for creating dopamine. Dr. Braverman has identified the following brain healthy foods as dopamine boosters:
  - Chicken (I recommend skinless)
  - Cottage cheese (I recommend 1% or fat-free)
  - Eggs (I recommend DHA-enriched eggs or egg whites)
  - Granola
  - Oat flakes (I recommend old-fashioned or steel-cut oats)
  - Ricotta cheese (I recommend low-fat)
  - Turkey (I recommend skinless)
  - Yogurt (I recommend low-fat and unsweetened)

- Higher-protein diets that are lower in simple carbohydrates (this means it's okay to eat the zucchini but not the zucchini muffins; okay to eat the carrots but not the carrot cake) tend to help this type.

- Exercise, especially doing an exercise you love, helps increase blood flow and dopamine in the brain. (See chapter 7 for more on which types of exercise are best for this type.)

- Focus by making a list of weight and health goals and put it where you can see it every day.

- Line up some outside supervision. Have someone you trust check in with you on a regular basis to help you stay focused.

- Avoid impulsively saying yes to offers for more food or drink and practice saying, "No, thank you, I'm full."

- From a supplement standpoint, green tea, rhodiola, and L-tyrosine are helpful.

- Stimulant medications—such as Adderall or Ritalin, which are commonly used to treat ADD, or phentermine—can be effective.

MEET GAYLE, AN IMPULSIVE OVEREATER

I met Gayle when she volunteered to come up on stage and get scanned when I appeared on *The Huckabee Show* with Governor Mike Huckabee. Gayle, thirty-nine, is 5′0″ (on a good day) and weighed 165 pounds. Before the show, she took our online questionnaire, which showed her to be an impulsive overeater. Before we went on air, we performed a QEEG test on her to measure electrical activity in the brain. Gayle's QEEG showed excessive theta, or slow, brain wave activity in the front part of her brain, confirming her brain pattern.

When I asked her about herself, she gave me the classic history for having lifetime ADD. She was distracted, off task, disorganized, and impulsive. She worked as a meeting planner and was constantly on the go. Years before, she had her colon removed because she had ulcerative colitis. She also had low thyroid, sleep apnea, and was a survivor of ovarian cancer and six rounds of chemotherapy. Certainly the low thyroid, sleep apnea, and chemotherapy could be the cause of the low activity we found in her brain, but Gayle said the ADD symptoms were present in childhood. She had even brought up the issue of ADD with her therapist, who dismissed it as being part of a creative personality.

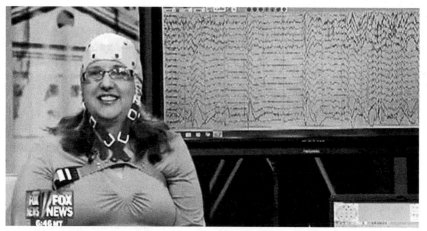

Gayle, a Type 2 Impulsive Overeater, on *The Huckabee Show* wearing a QEEG cap that measures electrical activity in the brain

The problem is that if you have low activity in your PFC you cannot be consistent with any nutritional plan or health program. You do not have the mental horsepower. Note that this does *not* mean that you are not intelligent enough—it just means that you don't have a PFC that is strong enough to put on the brakes when necessary.

Balancing her brain was critical to helping her be successful. The plan I gave Gayle included a diet higher in protein and lower in simple carbohydrates, which should help improve her focus. I also recommended that she write out clear goals, exercise at least four or five times a week, and take green tea and rhodiola. I told her that if the supplement was not strong enough to help her, then she should get treated for ADD with either a stimulant medicine, such as Adderall, or the appetite-suppressant phentermine.

Type 3. Impulsive-Compulsive Overeaters

GET SMART TO GET THINNER

"I found out I was a Type 3. Since I started balancing my brain, losing weight has become fun and easy. It's not a chore."

—Gina

People with this type have a combination of both impulsive and compulsive features. On the surface it seems almost contradictory. How can you be both impulsive and compulsive at the same time? Think of compulsive gambling. These are people who are compulsively driven to gamble and yet have very little control over their impulses. It is the same with these overeaters. Many people with bulimia also have this type.

These people often think about food all day long! For some, it can be 8:30 a.m., and they are already daydreaming about the beef-and-cheese lasagna they are going to have for dinner that night. Then, as they drive home from work on their way to that delectable meal, they pass by a fast-food restaurant and think, "Hey, some French fries would go really great with that lasagna. I'd better stop." The next thing they know, they have ordered not only a side of fries but also a bacon cheeseburger and a vanilla shake, which they devour in the car on the way home. Once they get home, they are no longer hungry but can't resist the lure of that cheesy lasagna that is waiting in the fridge. About 3,000 calories, 80 g saturated fat, and 100 g sugar later, they feel sick and disgusted with themselves and vow to do better tomorrow.

I have seen this type particularly common in children and grandchildren of alcoholics or people who have a significant family history of alcoholism. In the mid-1980s I noticed a connection between children and grandchildren of alcoholics and the combination of both impulsivity and compulsivity. My first wife grew up in an abusive alcoholic home. As a way to understand her better I started to research children of alcoholics. My work with brain SPECT helped me to understand this pattern further and we often saw increased ACG activity with lower PFC activity. Many of these patients did great on a combination of medications or supplements to raise both serotonin and dopamine.

Cherrie had bulimia as a teenager, and at age fifty-two she still struggled with bingeing and purging whenever she was stressed. She was chronically 30 pounds overweight and hated how she looked. She vacillated between being obsessive about her housework to being overwhelmed and disorganized. Many people in her family struggled with alcohol and other addictions. Cherrie had tried a number of diets without any success, until the fen-phen craze of the 1990s. Remember fen-phen? It was a combination of medications that increased both serotonin and dopamine. She did really well on it, losing 30 pounds, and felt more emotionally stable than at any time in her life. When fen-phen was pulled from the market because it caused medical problems, Cherrie relapsed and went back on her emotional and weight roller coaster. Without a balanced brain, she could not balance her weight.

Finally, Cherrie came to see us for help. On treatment to raise both serotonin and dopamine levels, she felt much more emotionally balanced and consistently lost weight.

SPECT FINDINGS FOR IMPULSIVE-COMPULSIVE OVEREATERS

Our scans tend to show too much activity in the ACG, so people overthink and get stuck on negative thoughts, but they also have too little activity in the PFC so they have trouble putting on the brakes and saying no. The low activity in the PFC is likely due to low dopamine levels, and the high activity in the ACG is associated with low serotonin levels.

WHAT MAKES IMPULSIVE-COMPULSIVE OVEREATERS WORSE

Using serotonin or dopamine interventions by themselves usually makes the problem worse. For example:

- Using a serotonin medication or supplement helps to calm the compulsions but makes the impulsivity worse.
- Using a dopamine medication or supplement helps to lessen the impulsivity but increases the compulsive behaviors.

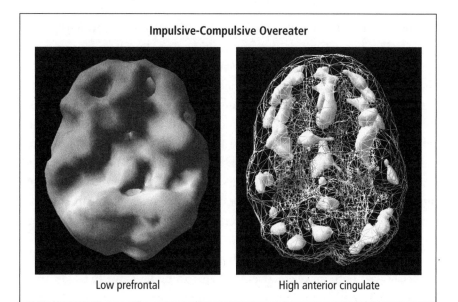

Impulsive-Compulsive Overeater

Low prefrontal | High anterior cingulate

WHAT WORKS FOR IMPULSIVE-COMPULSIVE OVEREATERS

In my experience, I have found that people with this type do best with treatments that raise both serotonin and dopamine. People with this mixed type tend to have done very well emotionally and behaviorally on the fen-phen combination, which raised both dopamine and serotonin in the brain. Plus, it is important to strengthen the PFC and practice strategies to help you get unstuck.

- Exercise. (See chapter 7 for more on which types of exercise are best for this type.)
- Set goals.
- Avoid automatically opposing others or saying no, even to yourself.
- Avoid impulsively saying yes.
- Have options.
- Distract yourself if you get a thought stuck in your head.
- From a supplement standpoint, combining green tea (for dopamine) and 5-HTP (for serotonin) can be helpful.
- When medications are necessary, combining phentermine (for dopamine) and Lexapro (for serotonin) may be effective.

MEET SHANICE, AN IMPULSIVE-COMPULSIVE OVEREATER

Shanice, thirty-three, always had a sweet tooth. As a child, she would sprinkle sugar on her Lucky Charms, put gummy bears and chocolate chips on top of her ice cream, and dip her toast in maple syrup. As an adult, her taste buds didn't change. She still craved sweets and would nibble on cookies on the way to work, munch on candy bars after lunch, and eat at least three scoops of ice cream late at night. Shanice was plagued by negative thoughts, and whenever she felt stressed she would turn to treats for comfort. The extra calories had added 40 pounds to her body, and she hated the way she looked. In her twenties, she developed bulimia in an effort to keep the weight off in spite of her overindulgences. Shanice came to see us to deal with her emotions following the death of her father, who had been an alcoholic for most of his life.

She had features of both impulsivity and compulsivity, and her SPECT scans showed both an overactive ACG and an underactive PFC. On treatment to raise both serotonin and dopamine, plus the behavioral strategies listed on page 116, Shanice finally got control of her cravings for sweets. Combined with psychotherapy, she was able to overcome her bulimia and finally lose weight and keep it off.

GET SMART TO GET THINNER

"My problems with eating started very, very young. If I could find a piece of bread, that's what I would eat to make painful feelings inside go away."

—Jeannie

Type 4. Sad or Emotional Overeaters

People with this type tend to use food to medicate underlying feelings of sadness and to calm the emotional storms in their brains. They often struggle with feelings of boredom, loneliness, depression, low self-esteem, and pain issues. Sad or emotional overeaters may also experience decreased libido, periods of crying, low energy levels, suicidal thoughts, and lack of interest in usually pleasurable activities, as well as feelings of guilt, helplessness, hopelessness, or worthlessness. For some people, these feelings come and go with the seasons and tend to worsen in winter. Others experience mild feelings of chronic sadness, called dysthymia. Still others suffer from more serious depressions. This type is more commonly seen in women.

SPECT FINDINGS FOR SAD OR EMOTIONAL OVEREATERS

The SPECT findings that correlate with this type are markedly increased activity in the deep limbic areas of the brain and decreased PFC activity. Treating mood disorders with behavioral interventions, natural supplements, and medication when needed, can be the key to weight loss.

When this type occurs in the winter, it is usually in more northern climates, where there is often a deficiency in sunlight and vitamin D levels. Having low levels of vitamin D, known as the "sunshine" vitamin, has been associated with depression, memory problems, obesity, heart disease, and immune suppression. Vitamin D deficiencies are becoming more common in our society for two reasons: We are wearing more sunscreen and we are spending more time indoors.

Some researchers believe nearly two-thirds of the U.S. population suffers from a vitamin D deficiency. I screen all of my patients for it by ordering a 25 hydroxy-vitamin D level. When we tested the vitamin D levels of more than thirty participants in our first weight-loss group, I was shocked to discover that everybody's levels were low, and this study took place in sunny Southern California!

WHAT MAKES SAD OR EMOTIONAL OVEREATERS WORSE

Certain behaviors can keep you mired in sadness, including:

- Letting yourself get stuck in negative thinking patterns
- Isolating yourself from friends and family
- Skimping on sleep

WHAT WORKS FOR SAD OR EMOTIONAL OVEREATERS

If you are a sad or emotional overeater, focus on activities and interventions that energize you and lift your mood.

- Exercise increases blood flow and multiple neurotransmitters in the brain and has been shown to be a mood booster. Several studies have found it to be as effective as antidepressant medication. (See chapter 7 for more on which types of exercise are best for this type.)

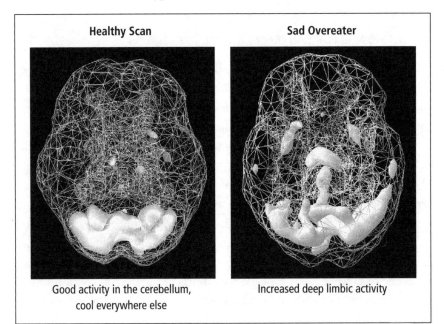

Healthy Scan	Sad Overeater
Good activity in the cerebellum, cool everywhere else	Increased deep limbic activity

- Kill the ANTs (automatic negative thoughts) that steal your happiness (more on this later).

- Write down five things you are grateful for every day. This has been shown to increase your level of happiness in just three weeks.

- Volunteer to help others, which helps to get you outside of yourself and less focused on your own internal problems.

- Surround yourself with great smells, such as lavender. This scent of lavender has been the subject of countless research studies, which show that it reduces cortisol levels and promotes relaxation and stress reduction.

- Try melatonin to help you sleep.

- Work to improve your relationships. Social bonding can help calm hyperactivity in the deep limbic system and enhance your mood.

- Increase your intake of omega-3 fatty acids by eating more fish, walnuts, avocados, and green leafy vegetables and/or taking a fish oil supplement (such as my Omega-3 Power). Low levels of omega-3 fatty acids have been associated with depression and obesity.

- Have your vitamin D levels checked and correct them if they are too low. Vitamin D supplements can help. Bright light therapy may also be helpful to correct vitamin D problems, help with mood states, and help people lose weight. There is evidence that bright light therapy might enhance the effectiveness of physical activity for weight loss. It significantly reduced the binge-eating episodes in people with bulimia and is an effective treatment for seasonal affective disorder (winter blues). It has even been shown to be more effective than Prozac for these patients. Using bright light therapy in the workplace was effective in improving mood, energy, alertness, and productivity.

- Check your DHEA blood levels. DHEA is a master hormone that has been found to be low in many people with depression and obesity. Supplementing with DHEA has good scientific evidence that it is helpful for weight loss in certain patients.

- Another helpful treatment for emotional overeaters is the natural supplement SAMe, in dosages of 400 to 1,600 mg. Be careful with SAMe if you have ever experienced a manic episode and take it early in the day as it has energizing properties and may interfere with sleep.

- If medication is necessary, I like Wellbutrin for this type, which has been shown to have weight-reducing properties.

MEET PAUL, A SAD OR EMOTIONAL OVEREATER

Paul was a supervisor at Boeing, located near Seattle. Over time he noticed that particularly in the winter, his weight would go up and his mood would go down. He struggled with depression for many years. Paul's problem wasn't a lack of willpower; it was his brain. His SPECT scan showed too much activity in the limbic or emotional part of his brain, which is commonly seen in mood disorders and in people who have had emotional trauma. Of note, Paul also had a very low vitamin D level, which has recently been associated with weight problems. For Paul, exercising and taking vitamin D, fish oil, and SAMe helped balance his brain, improve his mood, boost his energy, and keep the weight off in the winter.

Type 5. Anxious Overeaters

People with this type tend to medicate their feelings of anxiety, tension, nervousness, and fear with food. They tend to feel uncomfortable in their own skin. They may be plagued by feelings of panic, fear, and self-doubt, and suffer physical symptoms of anxiety, such as muscle tension, nail biting, headaches, abdominal pain, heart palpitations, shortness of breath, and sore muscles. It is as if they have an overload of tension and emotion. People with this type tend to predict the worst and often complain of waiting for something bad to happen. They may be excessively shy, easily startled, and freeze in emotionally charged situations.

SPECT FINDINGS FOR ANXIOUS OVEREATERS

The brain scans of anxious overeaters often show increased activity in the basal ganglia, which is commonly caused by low levels of the calming neurotransmitter GABA.

WHAT MAKES ANXIOUS OVEREATERS WORSE

Certain behaviors and substances can exacerbate feelings of anxiety and make you more likely to eat in an attempt to make those feelings go away. For example:

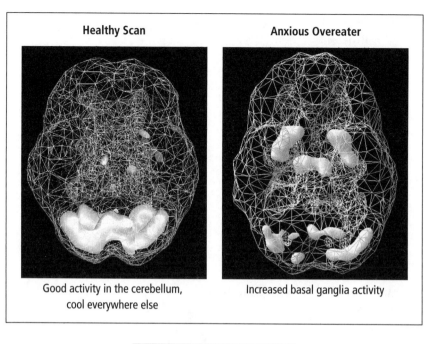

Healthy Scan	Anxious Overeater
Good activity in the cerebellum, cool everywhere else	Increased basal ganglia activity

GET SMART TO GET THINNER

"I ate to comfort and soothe my high anxiety."

—Sean

- Focusing on the negative
- Believing every negative thought you have
- For some anxious overeaters, consuming too much caffeine or other stimulating substances
- Drinking alcohol

WHAT WORKS FOR ANXIOUS OVEREATERS

Interventions to boost GABA combined with relaxation techniques that calm the brain are generally the most helpful. As with Type 4 Sad or Emotional Overeaters, many of the people who followed my home study course on overcoming anxiety and depression found that using the strategies to calm anxiety led to significant weight loss.

- Eat brain healthy foods that are high in the amino acid glutamine, a precursor to GABA. Dr. Braverman has identified the following brain healthy foods as being rich in GABA.

- Bananas
- Broccoli
- Brown rice
- Citrus fruit
- Halibut
- Herbal teas
- Lentils
- Nuts
- Oatmeal
- Spinach
- Whole grains

- Exercise. (See chapter 7 for more on which types of exercise are best for this type.)
- Try relaxation techniques, such as:
  - Meditation
  - Prayer
  - Hypnosis
  - Deep diaphragmatic breathing exercises
  - Hand-warming techniques

- Kill the anxious ANTs.
- For sleep, try self-hypnosis, kava kava, or valerian root.
- Vitamin B$_6$, magnesium, lemon balm, and GABA boost GABA in the brain.
- From a medication standpoint, the anticonvulsant Topamax has strong evidence it is helpful for weight loss, and in my experience, it is especially helpful for this type.

MEET CONNIE, AN ANXIOUS OVEREATER

Connie felt nervous most of the time. She was always waiting for something bad to happen—anticipating that her husband might get in a car accident or that she might get cancer. She frequently suffered from headaches and stomach problems. Marijuana helped relax her, but she hated doing something illegal. Food worked very well to calm her down, but being 5′2″ and 165 pounds made her very unhappy.

Connie's SPECT study showed too much activity in the basal ganglia. For Connie, no diet would help her lose weight until her brain was better. By soothing Connie's brain with meditation and hypnosis, plus using a combination of B_6, magnesium, and GABA (found in GABA Calming Support), she felt more relaxed and stopped overeating. She lost 20 pounds over the next year without trying and noticed a big boost in her energy.

The Amen Solution All-Stars: Eileen

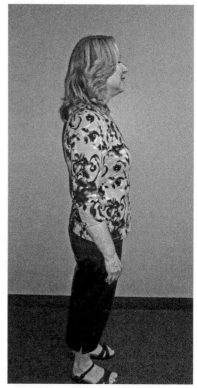

Before, 187 pounds

After three ten-week cycles,
lost 39 pounds

Eileen was so excited about her weight loss after participating in our program that she agreed to appear with me on *The Rachael Ray Show* to talk about her success. When Eileen joined the group, she weighed 187 pounds. By the end of the ten-week program, she had lost more than 15 pounds. She loved the program so much she took it again . . . and again. After twenty weeks, she had lost 26 pounds, and by the end of her third weight-loss cycle, she had lost 39 pounds, bringing her to 148 pounds. Since starting the program, she has gone down a total of *five* pant sizes.

When she took our questionnaire, she discovered that she was a Type 5 Anxious Overeater. She used food to comfort her and soothe her anxiety. Knowing this helped her focus on reducing her anxiety so she could finally lose some weight.

For Eileen, the most valuable part of the program was the *Daily Journal.* "I found the whole journal so helpful," she said. "It helps me think about the things I'm grateful for and helps me keep track of exercise. I can look at my day and say, 'Oh, here I blew it, but I can do better tomorrow.' Plus it has made me so much more thoughtful about what I choose to eat and more aware of what I'm eating. I had no idea how often I was eating without even realizing it and without really enjoying it."

She found that the *Daily Journal* helped keep her honest about her food intake. Tracking her calories also revealed something unexpected. She discovered that she would go long stretches without eating, which resulted in low blood sugar levels. As she learned in the weight-loss group, having low blood sugar can heighten feelings of anxiety and lower activity in the PFC, a combination that can lead to poor eating decisions. Eating more frequently throughout the day has helped her make better choices, like when she recently went to one of those huge buffets in Las Vegas. "I ate much healthier than I would have before," she said. "I don't even get tempted as much anymore by the things that aren't brain healthy."

Eileen used to reach for sweets when she felt anxious, but now she has so much less stress that the cravings for cookies, ice cream, and pie aren't really there anymore. Plus she has learned how to enjoy her favorite flavors in a healthier way by making simple food swaps. Here's how she does it: "I just put a little cinnamon and stevia on apples and it tastes like apple pie. I put powdered egg whites, stevia, frozen strawberries, and water in the blender and it tastes like a strawberry shake. I have pecans and a little unsweetened coconut and it tastes like pecan pie. Of course, I measure everything out to make sure I'm staying within my calorie limit."

For Eileen, the journal also served as a daily reminder to practice anxiety-reducing techniques, such as talking back to her ANTs. And like many Type 5 Anxious Overeaters, Eileen had a *lot* of ANTs. "I used to think I wasn't good enough," she admitted. "But thanks to the daily reminders, I kill my ANTs every day. It has become an automatic part of my day. My thinking has really changed. Having positive thoughts helps me get rid of my ANTs and reduce my anxiety."

Do You Have More Than One Type?

Having more than one type is common. For example, Type 3 Impulsive-Compulsive Overeaters is actually a combination of Type 1 Compulsive Overeaters and Type 2 Impulsive Overeaters. When you have more than one type, it just means that you may need a combination of interventions. With some combinations, you may only need to use the dominant treatment rather than trying to treat both types.

To help you understand which interventions are best if you have more than one type, I have created the following matrix. Of course, it is always smart to discuss these options with your health care provider. If he or she does not know much about natural treatments, consult a naturopath or a physician trained in integrative medicine or natural treatments.

If you have:	Use:
Types 1, 4	Type 1 interventions
Types 1, 5	Type 1 interventions
Types 1, 4, 5	Type 1 interventions
Types 2, 4	Type 2 interventions
Types 2, 5	Types 2 and 5 interventions
Types 2, 4, 5	Types 2 and 5 interventions
Types 3, 4	Type 3 interventions
Types 3, 5	Type 3 interventions
Types 3, 4, 5	Type 3 interventions
Types 4, 5	Types 4 and 5 interventions

SUMMARY TABLE OF THE FIVE TYPES OF OVEREATERS

Type	Symptoms	Brain Findings/ Neurotransmitter Issue	Supplements	Medications
1. Compulsive Overeaters	Overfocused on food, worrying, have trouble letting go of hurts	Increased AC (anterior cingulate)/low serotonin	5-HTP, inositol, saffron, or St. John's wort	SSRIs, such as Prozac, Zoloft, or Lexapro
2. Impulsive Overeaters	Impulsive, bored, easily distracted	Low PFC (prefrontal cortex)/ low dopamine	Green tea, rhodiola, L-tyrosine	Phentermine, or stimulants such as Adderall or Ritalin
3. Impulsive-Compulsive Overeaters	Combination of types 1 and 2	High AC plus low PFC/low serotonin and dopamine	5-HTP plus green tea and rhodiola	SSRI plus phentermine or stimulant
4. Sad or Emotional Overeaters	Sad or depressed mood, gets the winter blues, has carbohydrate cravings, loses interest, sleeps a lot, has low energy	High limbic activity/low PFC; check vitamin D and DHEA levels	SAMe, vitamin D, or DHEA if needed	Wellbutrin
5. Anxious Overeaters	Is anxious, tense, nervous; predicts the worst; eats to calm	High basal ganglia/ low GABA levels	GABA, B_6, magnesium	Topamax

5

TAKE BRAIN HEALTHY SUPPLEMENTS

LOSE WEIGHT, IMPROVE YOUR MOOD, AND RAISE YOUR IQ

If you are overweight, you have probably gazed longingly at those ads for "miracle drugs" that melt fat away. I hate to be the bearer of bad news, but there is no pill that is going to do all the work for you. Supplements will never work by themselves if you eat too much or do not exercise. What natural supplements *can* do, however, is help optimize your brain so it will be easier for you to be able to follow a brain healthy program.

Some supplements are so vital to brain health that I recommend them for everybody regardless of brain type. Other supplements are best geared to specific brain types to help balance those brains. Taking the right supplements for your brain type can jump-start your quest to be thinner, smarter, and happier.

Before I go into detail about each supplement, let me explain why I advocate their use. In treating people, one question I always ask myself is, what would I prescribe if you were my mother, my wife, or my child? More and more, after nearly thirty years of being a psychiatrist, I find myself recommending natural treatments. I am not opposed to medications, and I have prescribed them for a long time, but I want you to use all of the tools available, especially if they are effective, less expensive, and have fewer side effects.

One of the cases that got me interested specifically in natural treatments involved my own niece. When she was seven my sister brought her to see me for problems with moodiness and her temper. I tried her on a number of medications without any success. My sister was calling me, upset, three times a week. I kept using stronger and stronger medicines. But medications are not without risks and side effects, and when my niece started to gain weight I stopped them and decided to try her on a group of natural supplements that I had heard about from a colleague.

GET SMART TO GET THINNER

"It's so amazing to finally discover that the reason you can't lose weight isn't because you aren't trying hard enough, it's because your brain needs a little help."

—Rob

One day about four months later I realized that I hadn't heard anything from my sister in a long time. So I called her and said, "Hey, don't you love me anymore? How's my niece?"

She said, "Danny, you cannot believe the difference in her. She is so much better. She is calmer, more compliant, and she is getting straight As in school." The supplements have had long-term benefits for her without any side effects.

Pros and Cons of Supplements

Over time it made sense to start with natural supplements and then use medicines if the supplements didn't work. So, let's talk about the pros and cons of using natural supplements to help the brain. To start, they are often effective. They usually have dramatically fewer side effects than most prescription medications and they are significantly less expensive. Plus, you never have to tell an insurance company that you have taken them. As awful as it sounds, taking prescription medications can affect your insurability. I know many people who have been denied or made to pay higher rates for insurance because they have taken certain medications. If there are natural alternatives, they are worth considering.

GET SMART TO GET THINNER

"I just took it for granted that my brain was okay. I had never really thought about it before. But now I understand that I need to balance my brain."

—Sherri

Yet natural supplements also have their own set of problems. Even though they tend to be less expensive than medications, they may be more expensive for you because they are usually not covered by insurance. Many people are unaware that natural supplements can have side effects and need to be thoughtfully used. Just because something is natural does not mean it is innocuous. Both arsenic and cyanide are natural, but that doesn't mean they are good for you. For example, St. John's Wort, one of my favorite natural antidepressants, can cause sun sensitivity and it can also decrease the effectiveness of a number of medications, including birth control pills. Oh, great! Get depressed, pick up some St. John's Wort from the grocery store, and now you're accidentally pregnant. Not a good thing.

One of the major concerns about natural supplements is the lack of quality control. There is variability and you need to find brands you trust. Another disadvantage is that many people get their advice about supplements from the teenage clerk at the health food store who may not have the best information. But, even when looking at the problems, the benefits of natural supplements make them worth considering, especially if you can get thoughtful, research-based information.

Every day I personally take a handful of supplements that I believe make a significant difference in my life. They have helped to change the health of my brain, my energy, and my lab values. Many physicians say that if you eat a balanced diet you do not need supplements. I love what Dr. Mark Hyman wrote in his book *The UltraMind Solution: Fix Your Broken Brain by Healing Your Body First*. He wrote that if people "eat wild, fresh, organic, local, non–genetically modified food grown in virgin mineral- and nutrient-rich soils that has not been transported across vast distances and stored for months before being eaten . . . and work and live outside, breathe only fresh unpolluted air, drink only pure, clean water, sleep nine hours a night, move their bodies every day, and are free from chronic stressors and exposure to environmental toxins," then it is possible that they might not need supplements. Because we live in a fast-paced society where we pick up food on the fly, skip meals, eat sugar-laden treats, buy processed foods, and eat foods that have been chemically treated, we could all use a little help from a multiple vitamin and mineral supplements.

Amen Clinic Supplements

At the Amen Clinics we make our own line of supplements that have taken over a decade to develop. The reason I developed this line was that I wanted my patients and my own family to have access to the highest-quality research-based supplements available. After I started recommending supplements to my patients they would go to the supermarket, drugstore, or health food store and have so many choices that they did not know what or how to choose. Plus, there is variability of quality in the supplements available.

Another reason I developed my own line was that the Amen Clinics sees a high population of people who have ADD. I realized if they did not get their supplements as they walked out the door, they would forget about it or procrastinate and not have started them by their next appointment.

Research shows the therapeutic benefit of using supplements in treating mild to moderate depression, insomnia, and cognitive impairment. I strongly recommend that when purchasing a supplement, you consult your health care practitioner to determine which supplements and dosages may be most effective for you. Our website (www.amenclinics.com) contains links to the scientific literature on many different supplements related to brain health, so you, as a consumer, can be fully informed on the benefits and risks involved. Please remember supplements can have very powerful effects on the body and caution should be used when combining them with prescription medications.

GET SMART TO GET THINNER

"I started taking a high-quality multivitamin plus the fish oil and vitamin D and reduced the amount of wine I was drinking. After just a few weeks, I'm already sleeping better and feeling more energetic."

—Noelle

Three Supplements for Everybody

There are three supplements I typically recommend to *all* of my patients because they are critical to optimal brain function: a multivitamin, fish oil, and vitamin D.

MULTIVITAMINS

According to recent studies, more than 50 percent of Americans do not eat at least five servings of fruits and vegetables a day, the minimum required to get the nutrition you need. I recommend that all of my patients take a high-quality multivitamin / mineral complex every day. In an editorial in the

Journal of the American Medical Association, researchers recommended a daily vitamin for everybody because it helps prevent chronic illness. In addition, people with weight-management issues often are not eating healthy diets and have vitamin and nutrient deficiencies. Moreover, research suggests that people who take a multiple vitamin actually have younger-looking DNA.

A 2010 study from Northumbria University tested their effects on 215 men between the ages of thirty and fifty-five. For the double-blind, placebo-controlled study, the men were tested on mental performance and asked to rate themselves on general mental health, stress, and mood. At the debut of the trial, there were no significant differences between the multivitamin group and the placebo group. When the participants were restested a little over one month later, the multivitamin group reported improved moods and showed better mental performance, helping participants be happier and smarter! Not only that, but the multivitamin group reported an improved sense of vigor, reduced stress, and less mental fatigue after completing mental tasks.

Another placebo-controlled study from Northumbria researchers tested the effects of multivitamins on eighty-one healthy children aged eight to fourteen. They found that the children who took multivitamins performed better on two out of three attention tasks. The researchers concluded that multivitamins have the potential to improve brain function in healthy children.

FISH OIL

For years, I have been writing about the benefits of omega-3 fatty acids, which are found in fish oil supplements. I personally take a fish oil supplement every day and recommend that *all* of my patients do the same. When you look at the mountain of scientific evidence, it is easy to understand why. Research has found that omega-3 fatty acids are essential for optimal brain and body health.

GET SMART TO GET THINNER

"Now that I have learned about omega-3 fatty acids, I tell all the people I work with that it's important for them to take their fish oil."

—Liz

For example, according to researchers at the Harvard School of Public Health, having low levels of omega-3 fatty acids is one of the leading preventable causes of death and has been associated with heart disease, strokes, depression, suicidal behavior, ADD, dementia, and obesity. Scientific evidence also points to a link between low levels of omega-3 fatty acids and substance abuse. In my experience, I have found that *overeating is a form of substance abuse.*

I can tell you that most people, unless they are focusing on eating fish or taking fish oil supplements, have low omega-3 levels. I know this because at the Amen Clinics we perform a blood test on patients that measures their levels of omega-3 fatty acids. Before I began offering the test to patients, I tested it on my employees, several family members, and of course, myself. When my test results came back, I was very happy with the robust numbers. An omega-3 score above 7 is good. Mine was nearly 11. But the results for nearly all of the employees and family members I tested were not so good. In fact, I was horrified at how low their levels were, which put them at greater risk for both physical and emotional problems. It is an easy fix. They just needed to eat more fish or take fish oil supplements.

Boosting your intake of omega-3 fatty acids is one of the best things you can do for your brainpower, mood, and weight. The two most studied omega-3 fatty acids are eicosapentaenoic acid (EPA) and docosahexaenoic acid (DHA). DHA makes up a large portion of the gray matter of the brain. The fat in your brain forms cell membranes and plays a vital role in how our cells function. Neurons are also rich in omega-3 fatty acids. EPA improves blood flow, which boosts overall brain function.

How fish oil helps make you thinner. Increasing omega-3 intake has been found to decrease appetite and cravings and reduce body fat. In a fascinating 2009 study in the *British Journal of Nutrition,* Australian researchers analyzed blood samples from 124 adults (twenty-one healthy weight, forty overweight, and sixty-three obese), calculated their BMI, and measured their waist and hip circumference. They found that obese individuals had significantly lower levels of EPA and DHA compared with healthy-weight people. Subjects with higher levels were more likely to have a healthy BMI and waist and hip measurements.

More evidence about the benefits of fish oil on weight loss comes from a 2007 study from the University of South Australia. The research team found that taking fish oil combined with moderate exercise, like walking for forty-five minutes three times a week, leads to a significant reduction in body fat after just twelve weeks. But taking fish oil without exercising, or exercising without fish oil, did not result in any reduction in body fat.

One of the most intriguing studies I have found on fish oil and weight loss appeared in a 2007 issue of the *International Journal of Obesity.* In this study, researchers from Iceland investigated the effects of seafood and fish oils on weight loss in 324 young overweight adults with BMIs ranging from 27.5 to 32.5. The participants were placed in four groups that ate 1,600-calorie diets that were the same except that each group's diet included only one of the following:

- Control group (sunflower oil capsules, no seafood or fish oil)
- Lean fish group (3 × 150 g portions of cod per week)
- Fatty fish group (3 × 150 g of salmon per week)
- Fish oil group (DHA/EPA capsules, no seafood)

After four weeks, the average amount of weight loss among the men in each of the four groups was as follows:

- Control group: 7.8 pounds
- Lean fish group: 9.6 pounds
- Fatty fish group: 9.9 pounds
- Fish oil group: 10.9 pounds

The researchers concluded that adding fish or fish oil to a nutritionally balanced calorie-restricted diet could boost weight loss in men.

How fish oil helps make you happier. Research in the last few years has also revealed that diets rich in omega-3 fatty acids help promote a healthy emotional balance and positive mood in later years, possibly because DHA is a main component of the brain's synapses. A growing body of scientific evidence indicates that fish oil helps ease symptoms of depression. One twenty-year study involving 3,317 men and women found that people with the highest consumption of EPA and DHA were less likely to have symptoms of depression.

How fish oil helps make you smarter. There is a tremendous amount of scientific evidence pointing to a connection between the consumption of fish that is rich in omega-3 fatty acids and cognitive function. A Danish team of researchers compared the diets of 5,386 healthy older individuals and found that the more fish in a person's diet, the longer the person was able to maintain their memory and reduce the risk of dementia. Dr. J. A. Conquer and colleagues from the University of Guelph in Ontario, Canada, studied the blood fatty acid content in the early and later stages of dementia and noted low levels when compared with healthy people's. In 2010 UCLA researchers analyzed the existing scientific literature on DHA and fish oil and concluded that supplementation with DHA slows the progression of Alzheimer's and may prevent age-related dementia.

Omega-3 fatty acids benefit cognitive performance at every age. Scientists at the University of Pittsburgh reported in 2010 that middle-aged people with higher DHA levels performed better on a variety of tests, including nonverbal reasoning, mental flexibility, working memory, and vocabulary. In a study from Swedish researchers, results showed that surveyed nearly five thousand fifteen-year-old boys and found that those who ate fish more than once a week scored higher on standard intelligence tests than teens who ate no fish. A follow-up study found that teens eating fish more than once a week also had better grades at school than students with lower fish consumption.

Additional benefits of omega-3 fatty acids include increased attention in people with ADD, reduced stress, and a lower risk for psychosis. When we put our retired football players on our fish oil supplements, many of them were able to decrease or completely eliminate their pain medications.

My recommendation for most adults is to take 1–2 g high-quality fish oil a day.

VITAMIN D

Vitamin D, also known as the "sunshine vitamin," is best known for building bones and boosting the immune system. But it is also an essential vitamin for brain health, mood, memory, and your weight. While classified as a vitamin, it is a steroid hormone vital to health. Low levels of vitamin D have been associated with depression, autism and psychosis, Alzheimer's disease, multiple sclerosis, heart disease, diabetes, cancer, and obesity. Unfortunately, vitamin D deficiencies are becoming more and more common, in part because we are spending more time indoors and using more sunscreen when we're outdoors.

GET SMART TO GET THINNER

"When I started taking vitamin D, the weight started coming off faster."

—Deniece

How vitamin D helps you get thinner. Did you know that when you don't have enough vitamin D, you feel hungry all the time, no matter how much you eat? That is because low levels of vitamin D interfere with the effectiveness of leptin, the appetite hormone that tells you when you are full. Research also shows that vitamin D insufficiency is associated with increased body fat. A 2009 study out of Canada found that weight and body fat were significantly lower in women with normal vitamin D levels than women with insufficient levels. It appears that extra fat inhibits the absorption of vitamin D. The evidence shows that obese people need higher doses of vitamin D than lean people to achieve the same levels.

One of the most interesting studies I have seen on vitamin D comes from researchers at Stanford Hospital and Clinics. They detailed how a patient was given a prescription for 50,000 IU weekly of vitamin D that was incorrectly filled for 50,000 IU daily instead of weekly. After six months, the patient's vitamin D level increased from 7, which is extremely low, to 100, which is at the high end of normal.

What I found really intriguing about this report was that the patient complained of a few side effects from the very high dosage, namely decreased appetite and significant weight loss. Of course, I am not advocating that you take more vitamin D than you need. But I think it shows that optimal levels of vitamin D may play a role in appetite control and weight loss.

This patient's story shows why it is so important to get your vitamin D level checked before and after treatment. That way, you will know if you are taking the right dosage, or if you need to adjust the dosage.

GET SMART TO GET THINNER

"I was taking 4,000 IUs of vitamin D a day, and my level only went up to 38. The doctor said that was in the normal range and it was okay, but I want it to be in the optimal range (50–90), so I am going to increase my daily dosage."

—Ed

How vitamin D helps make you smarter. Did you know that vitamin D is so important to brain function that its receptors can be found throughout the brain? Vitamin D plays a critical role in many of the most basic cognitive functions, including learning and making memories. These are just some of the areas where vitamin D affects how well your brain works, according to a 2008 review that appeared in the *FASEB Journal.*

The scientific community is waking up to the importance of vitamin D for optimal brain function. In the past few years, I have come across a number of studies linking a shortage of vitamin D with cognitive impairment in older men and women, as well as some suggesting that having optimal levels of the sunshine vitamin may play a role in protecting cognitive function. One such study in the *Journal of Alzheimer's Disease* found that vitamin D_3, the active form of vitamin D, may stimulate the immune system to rid the brain of beta amyloid, an abnormal protein that is believed to be a major cause of Alzheimer's disease. Vitamin D activates receptors on neurons in regions important in the regulation of behavior, and it protects the brain by acting in an antioxidant and anti-inflammatory capacity.

Another study conducted in 2009 by a team at Tufts University in Boston looked at vitamin D level in more than 1,000 elderly people over the age of sixty-five and its effect on cognitive function. Only 35 percent of the participants had optimal vitamin D levels; the rest fell in the insufficient or deficient categories. The individuals with optimal levels of vitamin D—50 nmol/L (nanomole per liter) or higher—performed better on tests of executive functions, such as reasoning, flexibility, and perceptual complexity. They also scored higher on attention and processing speed tests than their counterparts with supoptimal levels.

How vitamin D helps make you happier. When it comes to being happy, the scientific evidence is clear. The lower your vitamin D levels, the more likely you are to feel blue rather than happy. Low levels of vitamin D have long been associated with a higher incidence of depression. In recent years, researchers have been asking if, given this association, vitamin D supplementation can improve moods.

One trial that attempted to answer that question followed 441 overweight and obese adults with similar levels of depression for one year. The individuals took either a placebo or one of two doses of vitamin D: 20,000 IU per week or 40,000 IU per week. By year's end, the two groups that had taken the vitamin D showed a significant reduction in symptoms while the group taking the placebo reported no improvements. Other trials have reported similar findings.

The current recommended dose for vitamin D is 400 IU daily, but most experts agree that this is well below the physiological needs of most individuals and instead suggest 2,000 IU of vitamin D daily. I think it is very important to test your individual needs, especially if you are overweight or obese, since your body may not absorb the vitamin D as efficiently if you are heavier.

The Amen Clinics All-Stars: Susan

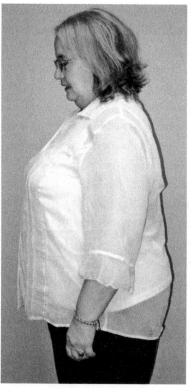 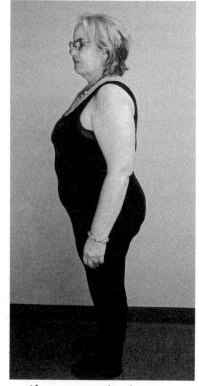

Before, 243 pounds

After two ten-week cycles, lost 29 pounds

Susan, fifty-nine, is just like so many of us. When she neared the age of thirty, she started putting on a few pounds, which didn't seem like much of a problem at the time. But then she continued to gain an extra 3 pounds a year for the next thirty years, bringing her to 243 pounds. Along the way, she tried dieting and would lose 20 pounds, but as soon as the diet was over, she'd gain it all back, and more. "They were all 'diets,'" she explained. "They weren't helping me understand my body."

When she learned about our brain-centered weight-loss program, she thought it might help her. "The whole brain approach really made sense to me because not everybody is the same. We're all different," she said. Learning about weight loss from a brain perspective was a completely new concept for her. "During the program, I kept having these 'aha' moments, like when Dr. Amen said, 'Don't drink your calories.' "

Susan used to have a glass of wine while preparing dinner, then another one or two with her meal and another one while she cleaned up. "Three or four glasses of wine—that's about 400 calories right there," she realized. Add to that the glasses of milk she liked to drink throughout the day, and she was easily drinking 600–700 calories a day.

Susan was very excited to figure out her brain type, but according to her answers, she didn't have one specific type. When this is the case, we typically recommend having someone else who knows you well complete the questionnaire for you. Many times, others are more honest and insightful about your behavior than you are. When that also reveals no specific type, we typically recommend the supplements that are beneficial for everyone regardless of brain type: a multivitamin, fish oil, and vitamin D. Having her important health numbers checked had revealed that Susan's vitamin D level was low, so supplementation was important for her. The first week she started taking vitamin D, she lost 7 pounds—in a single week. One thing that Susan's questionnaire did reveal was some trouble with her memory and "foggy thinking." So she started taking our Brain & Memory Power Boost and has noticed an improvement.

After a few weeks of learning about the brain and how it affects eating habits and weight, Susan started to reconsider some of her answers on the questionnaire and realized that perhaps she was more unfocused than she had originally indicated. "I think if I went back and took the questionnaire again, I would answer some of those questions differently. I feel like being unfocused was part of my problem," she said. "I just couldn't stay focused on doing the right thing." Because of this, she began taking our Focus & Energy Optimizer, which she says has helped her stay on track.

Stay on track is exactly what she has done. By keeping her meals to fewer than 500 calories each, preparing snacks whenever she goes out, and eliminating those high-calorie beverages, she has gotten her calories under control. In addition, she is now swimming three times a week and doing a meditation while she swims. In ten weeks, she lost 21 pounds. And unlike all those "diets" she had tried before, she has continued to lose weight after our ten-week program came to an end. "I've lost another 8 pounds and am on my way to my goal of getting under 200 pounds," she said.

Supplements That Support Craving Control

Anyone who has ever tried to lose weight knows that cravings can ruin your efforts and send you racing to the nearest pizza parlor, burger joint, or ice cream shop. Here, I will introduce you to natural supplements with scientific evidence showing that they can help take the edge off cravings. (See chapter 6 for more on this.)

ALPHA-LIPOIC ACID

Made naturally in the body, alpha-lipoic acid may protect against cell damage in a variety of conditions. There is strong evidence that alpha-lipoic acid supports stable blood sugar levels, which helps to decrease cravings and tendencies to overeat. Studies have shown that it improves insulin sensitivity and may be effective in treating type 2 diabetes. The typical recommended adult dose is 100 mg twice a day.

CHROMIUM

Chromium picolinate is a nutritional supplement used to aid the body in the regulation of insulin, which enhances its ability to efficiently metabolize glucose and fat. There is a strong link between depression, decreased insulin sensitivity, and diabetes. Supplementation with chromium picolinate has been shown to effectively modulate carbohydrate cravings and appetite, which is beneficial to managing both the diabetes and depression.

GET SMART TO GET THINNER

"When it comes to supplements, knowing your brain type is so important because if your brain needs serotonin to calm down and you take supplements that do the opposite, it makes it harder for you to succeed."

—Jimmy

I often recommend chromium picolinate to help with insulin regulation and to control carb cravings. In a well-designed study, 600 mcg (micrograms) chromium picolinate was beneficial for patients with atypical depression (the type of depression where people gain weight, rather than lose weight), especially those with carbohydrate cravings. Scientists at Oxford University in England demonstrated with animals that supplementing the diet with chromium enhances the activity of neurochemicals associated with mood control within the brain.

It is believed that chromium may help raise serotonin levels by facilitating the transport of certain amino acids within the brain and central nervous system. This could explain why it is helpful in reducing cravings for refined carbohydrates, which also raise serotonin levels. The typical recommended adult dosage is 200 to 600 micrograms a day.

DL-PHENYLALANINE

This is an essential amino acid (cannot be produced by the body) and thus must be obtained through the diet. Phenylalanine is used in different biochemical processes to produce the neurotransmitters dopamine, norepinephrine, and epinephrine. There is evidence that phenylalanine can increase mental alertness, release hormones affecting appetite, and reduce drug and alcohol cravings.

There have been reports that DL-phenylalanine can promote high blood pressure in those predisposed to hypertension. Monitoring in the first few months on phenylalanine can detect blood pressure increases in the minority of people who will have this symptom. Phenylalanine can promote the cell division of existing malignant melanoma cells. If you have melanoma, or any other form of cancer for that matter, avoid phenylalanine. Persons who have phenylketonuria cannot use phenylalanine. This includes those born with a genetic deficiency that prevents them from metabolizing phenylalanine. The typical recommended starting dosage for adults is 500 mg a day. Then slowly work up to 1,500 mg a day.

GET SMART TO GET THINNER

"After starting on the supplements for my brain type, I lost 13 pounds in less than three weeks. It has been effortless. My cravings are gone, and my impulsive-compulsive eating behavior is gone."

—Brad

L-GLUTAMINE

L-glutamine is an amino acid that is important in the synthesis of the excitatory neurotransmitter glutamate and the inhibitor neurotransmitter GABA. It is also a nutrient for the brain as it is used for energy if the brain does not have enough glucose to function. Supplemental glutamine has been shown to decrease carbohydrate cravings. The typical adult dose is 500 mg three to four times a day.

N-ACETYL-CYSTEINE

N-acetyl-cysteine, or NAC, is an amino acid that is needed to produce glutathione, a very powerful antioxidant. NAC binds to and removes dangerous toxic elements within the cells, making it a molecule critical to brain health. Recently, NAC has been studied as a treatment for drug addiction, as it functions to restore levels of the excitatory neurotransmitter glutamate in the reward center of the brain. A growing body of research has found that NAC can reduce cravings for cocaine, heroin, and cigarettes and decrease the risk for relapse. Considering that some foods activate the same areas of the brain as cocaine, it may be that NAC can also be helpful in reducing food cravings.

Other research concludes that NAC shows promise for the treatment of compulsive behavior problems. This means it could be helpful for Type 1 Compulsive Overeaters as well as those with impulsive-compulsive eating disorders, such as bulimia. The typical adult dose is 600–1,200 mg twice a day to curb cravings.

Supplements Recommended for Type 1 Compulsive Overeaters

5-HTP

There is good scientific evidence that 5-HTP helps with weight loss, and in my experience, I have found that it works best for this type. It is an amino acid building block for serotonin, and using this supplement is another way to increase cerebral serotonin, which may help control stress, improve sleep, and increase mood. A number of double-blind studies have shown 5-HTP is as effective as antidepressant medication. In my experience, I have found it to be very helpful for some people as a sleep aid.

GET SMART TO GET THINNER

> "For years I took vitamins on and off, but never felt better. Within one week of taking 5-HTP, I could get up in the morning and feel happy and less stressed. I can stop myself from worrying, and my junk food cravings are diminishing."
>
> —Terri

This supplement helps to calm anterior cingulate gyrus hyperactivity (to help shift attention). For people who can't seem to turn off their brains at bedtime, or who have anxious thoughts that keep them awake, 5-HTP may help. The most common side effect of 5-HTP is an upset stomach, although it is usually mild. To avoid an upset stomach, start by taking small doses of 5-HTP and gradually increase the dosage as you get used to it. Taking it with food can also help. Because 5-HTP increases serotonin, you should not take it with other medications that increase serotonin, such as St. John's Wort, L-tryptophan, or prescribed antidepressants, unless you are closely supervised by your physician.

The typical adult dose of 5-HTP is 50–100 mg two or three times daily with or without food.

INOSITOL

Inositol is a sugar that is considered part of the B vitamin family. It is a natural chemical found in the brain that is reported to help neurons use serotonin more efficiently. It is important in the maintenance of cell membranes, the breakdown of fat, hair growth, and the regulation of estrogen and insulin. Studies demonstrate its efficacy in treating those with obsessive-compulsive disorder, panic disorder, and anxiety disorders. It also functions to neutralize free-radical activity, thereby protecting neurons and promoting brain health.

Scientific studies have shown that 12–18 g inositol daily has beneficial effects in the treatment of depression, anxiety, panic disorder, and obsessive-compulsive disorder.

L-TRYPTOPHAN

Scientific evidence shows that L-tryptophan can help people lose weight. Like 5-HTP, L-tryptophan is an amino acid building block for serotonin, and taking L-tryptophan supplements increases cerebral serotonin. Serotonin is a neurotransmitter that plays an important role in mood stabilization and sleep, as well as a number of other functions. The high doses of L-tryptophan found in turkey may explain why we get sleepy after devouring a big Thanksgiving meal.

L-tryptophan was taken off the market more than a decade ago because one contaminated batch from one manufacturer caused a rare blood disease and a number of deaths. L-tryptophan itself actually had nothing to do with these deaths. L-tryptophan was reapproved by the Food and Drug Administration several years ago and is currently available again. One of the problems with dietary L-tryptophan is that a significant portion of it does not enter the brain, but rather is used to make proteins and vitamin B_3. This necessitates taking large amounts of L-tryptophan.

The typical adult dose is 1,000–3,000 mg taken at bedtime.

SAFFRON

Saffron is grown in Iran, Greece, Spain, and Italy and traditionally has been used to ease the digestion of spicy food, to soothe an irritated stomach, and to treat depression. The saffron extract called satiereal is a patented product that has been shown to have antidepressant effects. The active ingredients of satiereal include safranal, picrocrocin, and crocin, which work synergistically to help with satiety and to help curb the compulsive desire to eat.

Like SSRIs, satiereal is thought to work by preventing the reuptake of serotonin, thereby improving mood and well-being. It differs in that a small amount is potent, and it has been shown to be a successful weight loss aid by reducing appetite and sugar cravings. In clinical trials satiereal has been shown to be well tolerated with few adverse side effects.

The recommended dosage is 100 mg twice a day.

GET SMART TO GET THINNER

"All my life I have been large. At eighteen months, I weighed 54 pounds. By the time I got to the eleventh grade, I weighed 310 pounds. As an adult, I got up to 445 pounds. I have tried most diet programs as well as diet pills. Nothing worked. But then I saw your public television special and read your book. Now it's no to fast food, no to soda pop, and yes to water aerobics twice a week. I started taking a multivitamin, vitamin D, fish oil, and 5-HTP. In less than six months, I have lost 89 pounds."

—Randy

ST. JOHN'S WORT

A plant located in the subtropical regions of North America, Europe, Asia, India, and China, St.-John's-wort *(Hypericum perforatum)* has been used for centuries in the treatment of mood disorders and depression. The biologically active ingredient in St. John's Wort is hypericin, which functions to inhibit the reuptake of various neurotransmitters including serotonin, dopamine, GABA, and glutamate. The mechanism of action for St. John's Wort is similar to that found in popular antidepressants, including Prozac, Paxil, and Zoloft. These drugs and the herb work to maintain elevated levels of serotonin, which has a mood-enhancing effect.

Stress depletes the brain of serotonin. St. John's Wort combats that and may actually be the most potent of all the supplements at increasing serotonin availability in the brain. I have seen dramatic improvement for many of my patients on St. John's Wort and have SPECT scan studies of patients before and after treatment with St. John's Wort that document its effectiveness. St. John's Wort decreases anterior cingulate gyrus hyperactivity (which can make you rigid and stressed out when things don't go your way) for many patients and decreases moodiness.

An unfortunate side effect is that it can also decrease prefrontal cortex activity. One of the women in a study we conducted said, "I'm happier, but I'm dingier." We also don't start people with temporal lobe symptoms (anger, epilepsy, memory problem, hallucinations, and so on) on St. John's Wort without first stabilizing the temporal lobes with anticonvulsant medication. An important note is that it has been found to decrease the effectiveness of other drugs, including birth control pills.

The typical dose is 300 mg a day for children, 300 mg twice a day for teens, and 600 mg in the morning and 300 mg at night for adults. Sometimes, the dose may be slowly increased to 1,800 mg for adults. It is important that the preparation of St. John's Wort contain 0.3 percent hypericin, which is believed to be one of the active ingredients of St. John's Wort.

Supplements Recommended for Type 2 Impulsive Overeaters

GREEN TEA LEAF EXTRACT

Made from the dried leaves of *Camellia sinensis,* green tea leaf extract is an evergreen shrub. It has been used as a remedy for many ailments, including anxiety, cancer prevention, and cardiovascular health; for the prevention of cold and flu; and for weight loss. The green tea component epigallocatechin gallate, often referred to as EGCG, is a potent free-radical scavenger. Included in the extract is L-theanine, which has been shown to enhance brain wave alpha states, and increase relaxation and focus. A 2009 study tested the effects of green tea leaf extract on weight loss. One hundred men and women were placed on a calorie-restricted diet with half of them receiving a green tea leaf extract supplement while the other half did not. After ninety days, the group taking the supplement had lost an average of 31 pounds compared with 11 pounds for the diet-only group.

GET SMART TO GET THINNER

"With the Focus & Energy Optimizer, which contains green tea and rhodiola, I don't need coffee in the afternoon anymore."

—Ty

The typical adult dose is 200–300 mg green tea leaf extract capsules daily for cancer prevention and possible effects on weight loss. Up to 3 cups a day of green tea can be consumed for health benefits, but caution should be used with pregnant women as green tea does contain caffeine.

L-TYROSINE

This amino acid is important in the synthesis of brain neurotransmitters. It is the precursor to the brain neurotransmitters epinephrine, norepinephrine, and dopamine, which are critical for balancing mood and energy. It is also helpful in the process of producing thyroid hormones, which are important in metabolism and energy production. A sluggish thyroid can have significant effects on brain health and can contribute to weight problems. The beneficial effect of tyrosine supplementation is that an efficiently functioning thyroid will not only result in a better-functioning brain but will also help in weight loss.

Tyrosine supplementation has been shown to improve cognitive performance under periods of stress and fatigue. Stress tends to deplete the neurotransmitter norepinephrine, and tyrosine is the amino acid building block to replenish it. Tyrosine should not be taken with MAO (monamine oxidase) inhibitors and tricyclic antidepressants, when a cancerous melanoma is present, with a history of cancerous melanoma, or with elevated blood pressure.

The typical adult dose is 500–1500 mg two to three times a day. It is best taken on an empty stomach with water or juice. Be cautious when taking DL-phenylalanine and L-tyrosine together, as they may be too stimulating.

RHODIOLA

An herb that is grown at high altitudes in Asia and Europe, rhodiola has traditionally been used to fight fatigue, improve memory, and increase attention span. It is called an adaptogen, because it helps plants adapt to harsh environments. Research has found that it does indeed help prevent fatigue. In addition, scientific evidence points to an ability to fuel sexual energy, boost immunity, and ease depression. In a study we conducted at the Amen Clinics with Dr. Mahtab Jafari from the University of California–Irvine, we found that rhodiola helped to increase blood flow to the brain, especially the prefrontal cortex. Our study group also reported better mood and energy.

The typical adult dose is 200–600 mg daily for the treatment of fatigue and depression and it is best taken on an empty stomach. Rhodiola should be taken early in the day as it may interfere with sleep and it should not be used in individuals with bipolar disorder or those taking hypertensive or hypoglycemic medications.

Supplements Recommended for
Type 3 Impulsive-Compulsive Overeaters

For this type, taking a combination of 5-HTP plus green tea leaf extract and rhodiola is best. (See descriptions above.)

GET SMART TO GET THINNER

"I used to always gain weight in the winter and lose it in the summer. I never realized it was because I was having the 'winter blues' and eating more as a way of dealing with those feelings. Taking the supplements helped me control my moods and my eating."

—Tamara

Supplements Recommended for
Type 4 Sad or Emotional Overeaters

Vitamin D and fish oil supplements are especially important for this type. (See descriptions above.)

SAMe

S-adenosyl methionine (SAMe) is involved in the production of several neurotransmitters (serotonin, dopamine, epinephrine) and helps the brain to function properly. The brain normally manufactures all the SAMe it needs from the amino acid methionine. When a person is depressed, the synthesis of SAMe from methionine is impaired, and SAMe has been shown to have antidepressant qualities. People who have a certain type of ADD that is linked with depression may experience an improvement in mood and focus when taking SAMe. SAMe has also been found to suppress appetite and reduce joint inflammation and pain.

The typical adult dose is 200–400 mg two to four times a day. Caution should be taken with people who have a tendency toward bipolar disorder. Usually, it is best to take early in the day as it may be stimulating for some.

DHEA

DHEA is a master hormone that has been found to be low in many people with depression and obesity. There is good scientific evidence that supplementing with DHEA is helpful for weight loss in certain patients. DHEA is one of the most abundant hormones in the body, second only to cholesterol. It is usually well tolerated. Acne and facial hair are common side effects, as it increases the body's testosterone levels. To avoid getting acne or facial hair, many doctors prescribe a metabolite of DHEA called 7-keto-DHEA. It is more expensive, but if acne and facial hair are an issue, it is worth it.

The main worry about DHEA by some professionals is that it will partly convert itself into sex hormones such as testosterone and estrogens. This seems to be an obvious advantage for healthy people who are looking to combat age-associated hormonal decline. Unfortunately, this means advising people who are at risk for hormonally dependent cancers (prostate, breast, ovarian) against taking DHEA. For these, 7-keto-DHEA is a good solution.

DHEA supplementation is not recommended for children, adolescents, and pregnant or nursing women. Androgenic effects including acne, hair loss, and a deepening of the voice have been reported in women. If this occurs, discontinue DHEA immediately.

The typical recommended adult dosage is 25–50 mg daily. DHEA is banned by the International Olympic Committee, the National Collegiate Athletic Association, the NFL, and other sports organizations for its performance-enhancing properties.

B VITAMINS

The B vitamins play an integral role in the functioning of the nervous system and help the brain synthesize neurotransmitters that affect mood and thinking. Some research indicates that supplementation with some of the B vitamins may fight depression. For example, a 2003 study out of Finland found that taking vitamin B_{12} might aid in the recovery from major depressive disorder. In 2010 researchers from Rush University Medical Center in Illinois reported that taking vitamins B_6 and B_{12} may reduce the risk of depression in older adults.

The typical adult dose of B_6 is 25–50 mg. For B_{12}, it is 250 mcg.

Supplements Recommended for Type 5 Anxious Overeaters

GABA

Gamma-aminobutyric acid (GABA) is an amino acid that also functions as a neurotransmitter in the brain. GABA is reported in the herbal literature to work in much the same way as anti-anxiety drugs and anticonvulsants. It helps stabilize nerve cells by decreasing their tendency to fire erratically or excessively. This means it has a calming effect for people who struggle with anxiety, irritability, or temper, whether these symptoms relate to anxiety or to temporal lobe disturbance.

GET SMART TO GET THINNER

"I used to grab for the bread or muffins whenever I felt anxious. Now that I'm taking the right supplements and doing my relaxation exercises, I don't have all that anxiety anymore and my bread cravings are gone."

—Emma

The typical recommended adult dosage ranges from 100 to 1,500 mg daily for adults and from 50 to 750 mg daily for children. For best effect, GABA should be taken in two or three doses a day.

MAGNESIUM

Magnesium is a mineral that is essential to good health as it is needed for more than three hundred biochemical reactions in the body. It has been shown to be helpful in calming anxiety and balancing the brain's pleasure centers, which can help reduce cravings. Magnesium is also important in energy production and assists in calcium and potassium uptake in the body. A deficiency in magnesium can lead to irritability and nervousness. Supplementing the body with magnesium can help with mood and muscle weakness. In combination with vitamin B_6, it has been shown to reduce the hyperactivity seen in children with ADD.

Scientists have long known that magnesium also plays an important role in memory and learning. Research in a 2010 issue of the journal *Neuron* indicates that increasing magnesium in the brain enhances learning abilities in children and adults. Not only that this vital nutrient improved working memory, short-term memory, and long-term memory. The researchers discovered that elevating magnesium levels created positive changes in the hippocampus, one of the brain's major memory centers.

The typical adult dose is 400–1,000 mg daily, divided into three doses. It is best to take with calcium as these minerals work synergistically. Magnesium is usually half of your total calcium intake.

VALERIAN ROOT

Many patients find valerian to be remarkably helpful as a sleeping aid and stress-relief aid. Since valerian promotes sleep, it may also help balance leptin and ghrelin, the appetite hormones that are regulated during sleep. When these hormones are balanced, they do a better job of telling you when you are full so you can stop overeating.

Valerian is a well-recognized herb with antianxiety properties that is used as a mild tranquilizer, sedative, and muscle relaxant. There are about 150 species of valerian widely distributed in temperate regions of the world. The active ingredient is found in a foul-smelling oil produced in the root of the plant. Throughout history, people have turned to valerian for its unique properties. The ancient Roman physician Galen wrote about the virtues of valerian; in the Middle Ages, medical literature used the term *All Heal* to describe the herb; and valerian has long been a staple of Chinese and Indian medicine. In the United States, valerian was commonly used prior to the development of modern pharmaceuticals.

This centuries-old treatment for insomnia has also been helpful for symptoms of nervousness, stress, and pain. It has also been found to decrease seizure frequency in epileptic patients. Studies have shown valerian to be helpful for many types of anxiety disorders and for people with performance anxiety and those who get stressed in daily situations like traffic. Valerian appears to work by enhancing the activity of the calming neurotransmitter, GABA.

Unlike prescription tranquilizers, valerian has no potential for addiction and has been used to help people who are trying to decrease their use of prescription tranquilizers or sleeping pills. (Anyone using prescription sleeping pills or tranquilizers should decrease or stop their use only under the supervision of a physician.) It may take two to three weeks to start feeling the effects of valerian, so it isn't the best sleep aid for short-term use, such as when you have jet lag. It is better suited for long-term use and has been found to improve deep sleep, which leaves you feeling more rested in the morning. Valerian should not be taken in combination with alcohol, barbiturates, or benzodiazepines, and it is not recommended for use during pregnancy or while breast-feeding.

Valerian is available in capsules, tablets, liquids, tinctures, extracts, and teas. Most extracts are standardized to 0.8 percent valeric acids. The typical recommended adult dosage is 150 to 450 mg in capsules or teas.

VITAMIN B$_6$

The B vitamins are especially effective in controlling stress. When you are faced with stressful situations or thoughts, the B vitamins are typically the first to be depleted. If you have a B-vitamin deficiency, your ability to cope with stress and anxiety is lowered. As you well know, it is much harder to say no to the pizza, cheesecake, and cinnamon rolls when you are under a lot of stress.

Vitamin B$_6$ (pyridoxine) is a water-soluble vitamin essential in the metabolism of amino acids, glucose, and fatty acids and is important in the production of neurotransmitters (serotonin, epinephrine, norepinephrine, and

GABA). It is required by the nervous system and is needed for normal brain function as well as DNA synthesis. It is hard to find a molecule in our bodies that doesn't rely on vitamin B_6 for its production. It is involved in more than one hundred crucial chemical reactions in our bodies.

Vitamin B_6 helps our nervous system function properly. It is required for the production of hemoglobin, the compound in red blood cells that transports oxygen and carbon dioxide. It increases the amount of oxygen carried in our blood, helping overcome fatigue. It helps maintain a healthy immune system and calms anxiety. It also helps in processing carbohydrates for energy. Food sources of vitamin B_6 include fortified cereals, beans, meat, poultry, fish, and some fruits and vegetables.

The typical adult dose of vitamin B_6 is 25 to 50 mg daily.

More Supplements That Make You Smarter

CHOLINE

This nutrient is essential to the structure and function of all cells. It is a precursor molecule involved in the synthesis of the neurotransmitter acetylcholine, which is important for normal brain function. Those deficient in acetylcholine may develop Alzheimer's disease and dementia; therefore, choline supplementation may be helpful in preventing the onset of these neurological disorders.

Choline is also involved in producing the cell membrane phospholipids phosphatidylcholine and sphingomyelin. The breakdown of cell membranes leads to neuronal death. Therefore, replenishing these vital components of the membrane is a proactive step you can take to help prevent Alzheimer's disease.

Food sources of choline include egg yolk, liver, peanuts, fish, milk, and cauliflower. Generally, up to 3 g choline daily is well tolerated, but possible side effects may include nausea, diarrhea, dizziness, sweating, and hypotension.

The recommended dosage is 300–1,200 mg daily.

GINKGO BILOBA

The prettiest brains I have seen are those on ginkgo. Ginkgo biloba, from the Chinese ginkgo tree, is a powerful antioxidant that is best known for its ability to enhance circulation, memory, and concentration. Consider taking ginkgo if you suffer from low energy or decreased concentration.

GET SMART TO GET THINNER

"A lot of people don't notice that their memory isn't as sharp as it used to be. It wasn't until I started doing this program and taking the vitamins, fish oil, vitamin D, and Brain & Memory Power Boost that I realized I wasn't as sharp as I wanted to be. Now my memory is improving."

—Phil

The best-studied form of ginkgo biloba is a special extract called EGb 761, which has been studied in blood-vessel disease, clotting disorders, depression, and Alzheimer's disease. A comparison in 2000 of all the published, placebo-controlled studies longer than six months for ginkgo biloba extract, EGb 761, versus Cognex, Aricept, and Exelon showed they all had similar benefits for mild to moderate Alzheimer's disease patients.

The most widely publicized U.S. study of ginkgo biloba appeared in the *Journal of the American Medical Association* in 1997 and was conducted by Dr. P. L. Le Bars and colleagues from the New York Institute for Medical Research. EGb 761 was used to assess its efficacy and safety in Alzheimer's disease and vascular dementia. It was a fifty-two-week multicenter study with patients who had mild to severe symptoms. Patients were randomly assigned to treatment with EGb 761 (120 mg per day) or placebo. Progress was monitored at twelve, twenty-six, and fifty-two weeks, and 202 patients finished the study. At the end of the study, the authors concluded that EGb 761 was safe and appears capable of stabilizing and, in a substantial number of cases, improving the cognitive performance and the social functioning of demented patients for six months to one year. Although modest, the changes induced by EGb were objectively measured and were of sufficient magnitude to be recognized by the caregivers. Other large-scale studies have not found a positive benefit. Our experience is that gingko does enhance blood flow to the brain.

In a double-blind placebo-controlled study from Brazil in 2003 using SPECT, researchers studied 48 men between the ages of 60 and 70 for eight months and found significant improvements in blood flow and global cognitive functioning for those taking gingko, while the placebo group showed the opposite with decreased brain blood flow and poorer scores on cognitive testing.

Consider taking ginkgo if you are at risk for memory problems or stroke or if you suffer from low energy or decreased concentration. There is a small risk of bleeding in the body, and the dosages of other blood-thinning agents being taken may sometimes need to be reduced.

The typical adult dose is 60 to 120 mg twice daily.

HUPERZINE A

This remarkable compound has been studied in China for nearly twenty years. It appears to work by increasing the availability of acetylcholine, a major memory neurotransmitter in the brain, and preventing cell damage from excitotoxins. It has been shown to be effective in improving patients who suffered with cognitive impairment from several different types of dementia, including Alzheimer's disease and vascular dementia. Since 1991 it has been studied as a treatment for the prevention of Alzheimer's disease and can be considered safe to use as an alternative or adjunct to medication in the treatment of Alzheimer's disease.

Huperzine A has also been found to help learning and memory in teenagers. Researchers divided thirty-four pairs of junior high school students complaining of memory problems into a Huperzine A group and a placebo control group. The Huperzine A group was given two (50 mcg) capsules of Huperzine A twice a day, while the placebo group was given two capsules of placebo (starch and lactose inside) twice a day for four weeks. At the end of the trial, the Huperzine A group's memory abilities were significantly superior to that of the placebo group.

Those with seizure disorders, cardiac arrhythmias, asthma, or irritable bowel syndrome should talk to their health care professionals before taking Huperzine A. Possible side effects include headaches, gastrointestinal effects, dizziness, blurred vision, slow heart rate, arrhythmias, seizures, and increased urination. Use of Huperzine A with acetylcholinesterase inhibitors or cholinergic drugs may produce additive effects, so caution should be used.

The typical adult dose is 50–100 mcg twice a day and 200–400 mcg daily if cognitive impairment is already noted.

PHOSPHATIDYLSERINE

Phosphatidylserine (PS) is a naturally occurring nutrient that is found in foods such as fish, green leafy vegetables, soy products, and rice. PS is a component of cell membranes. As we age, these membranes change in composition. There are reports of the potential of PS to help improve age-related declines in memory, learning, verbal skills, and concentration. PS is essential to brain health by maintaining neurons and neuronal networks so that the brain can continue to form and retain memories.

PET (positron emission tomography) studies of patients who have taken PS show that it produces a general increase in metabolic activity in the brain. In the largest multicenter study to date of phosphatidylserine and Alzheimer's disease, 142 subjects aged forty to eighty were given 200 mg PS per day or placebo over a three-month period. Those treated with PS exhibited improvement on several items on the scales normally used to assess Alzheimer's status. The differences between placebo and experimental groups were small but statistically significant.

The types of symptoms that have improved in placebo-controlled studies of cognitive impairment or dementia include loss of interest, reduced activities, social isolation, anxiety, and loss of memory, concentration, and recall. Milder stages of impairment tend to respond to PS better than more severe stages. With regard to depression in elderly individuals, Dr. M. Maggioni and colleagues studied the effects of oral PS (300 mg per day) versus placebo and noted significant improvements in mood, memory, and motivation after thirty days of PS treatment.

In a 2010 study from Israel, researchers evaluated the efficacy of PS plus DHA (PS-DHA) in 157 nondemented elderly people with memory complaints. The group participants received either PS-DHA or placebo for 15 weeks. Efficacy was measured following 7 and 15 weeks of treatment. Verbal immediate recall was significantly improved in the PS-DHA group compared with the placebo group.

PS has also been reported to be helpful for adrenal fatigue. The typical adult dose is 100–300 mg a day.

SAGE

NaturalStandard.com gives the common herb sage its highest "A level" scientific evidence rating for cognitive improvement. It cites research that has demonstrated that sage can improve memory, confirming centuries-old theories. In the seventeenth century noted herbalist Nicholas Culpeper wrote that the herb sage could "heal" the memory while "warming and quickening the senses."

Culpeper wasn't the only herbalist (and certainly not the first) to recognize that sage can help improve memory. Now—centuries later—scientists believe they know why. An enzyme called acetylcholinesterase (AChE) breaks down a chemical called acetylcholine that is typically deficient in Alzheimer's patients. Researchers from the Medical Plant Research Centre (MPRC) at the Universities of Newcastle and Northumbria in the United Kingdom have shown that sage inhibits AChE.

A study conducted by researchers at MPRC demonstrates the possible results of inhibiting AChE. Researchers gave forty-four subjects either sage oil capsules or placebo capsules containing sunflower oil and then conducted word recall tests. The group that received sage oil turned in significantly better test results than subjects who took placebo. However, researchers say that further tests are needed to fully determine just how far-reaching sage's effect may be on memory.

The typical adult dose for improved mood, alertness, and cognitive performance is 300–600 mg daily of dried sage leaf capsules. Sage can also be used as an essential oil in doses of 25 to 50 mcL (microliters). Sage should be used cautiously in those with hypertension or those who have seizure disorders.

VINPOCETINE

This brain booster is sometimes called a nootropic, or cognition enhancer, from the Greek word *noos* for "mind." Vinpocetine has been shown in a number of studies to help memory, especially for people who are at risk for heart disease or strokes. It also helps lower high homocysteine levels, which are also dangerous to your heart and brain.

Vinpocetine is derived from an extract of the common periwinkle plant *(Vinca minor)* and is used in Europe, Japan, and Mexico as a pharmaceutical agent for the treatment of blood-vessel disease in the brain and cognitive disorders. In the United States it is available as a dietary supplement.

Vinpocetine selectively widens arteries and capillaries, increasing blood flow to the brain. It also combats accumulation of platelets in the blood, improving circulation. Because of these properties, vinpocetine was first used in the treatment of cerebrovascular disorders and acute memory loss owing to late-life dementia. But it also has a beneficial effect on memory problems associated with normal aging.

There is evidence that vinpocetine may be useful for a wide variety of brain problems. A 1976 study found that vinpocetine immediately increased circulation in fifty people with abnormal blood flow. After one month of taking moderate doses of vinpocetine, patients showed improvement on memorization tests. After a prolonged period of vinpocetine treatment, cognitive impairment diminished significantly or disappeared altogether in many of the patients. A 1987 study of elderly patients with chronic cerebral dysfunction found that patients who took vinpocetine performed better on psychological evaluations after the ninety-day trial period than did those who received a placebo.

GET SMART TO GET THINNER

"Yes, I'm losing weight, but I'm also in a better mood and don't get so angry anymore."

—Miguel

More-recent studies have shown that vinpocetine reduces neural damage and protects against oxidative damage from harmful beta-amyloid buildup. In a multicenter double-blind placebo-controlled study lasting sixteen weeks, 203 patients described as having mild to moderate memory problems, including primary dementia, were treated with varying doses of vinpocetine or placebo. Significant improvement was achieved in the vinpocetine-treated group as measured by "global improvement" and cognitive performance scales. Three 10-mg doses daily were as effective or more effective than three 20-mg doses daily.

Similarly good results were found in another double-blind clinical trial testing vinpocetine versus placebo in elderly patients with blood vessel and central nervous system degenerative disorders. Some preliminary research suggests that vinpocetine may also have some protective effects in both sight and hearing.

Reported adverse reactions include nausea, dizziness, insomnia, drowsiness, dry mouth, transient hypotension, transient fast heart rate, pressure headaches, and facial flushing. Slight reductions in both systolic and diastolic blood pressure with prolonged use of vinpocetine have been reported, as well as slight reductions in blood sugar levels.

The typical adult dose is 10 mg a day.

Supplements That Help You Get Better Sleep

MELATONIN

Melatonin is a hormone made in the brain that helps regulate other hormones and maintains the body's sleep cycle. Darkness stimulates the production of melatonin while light decreases its activity. Exposure to too much light in the evening or too little light during the day can disrupt the production of melatonin. Jet lag, shift work, and poor vision are some of the conditions that can disrupt melatonin production. Some researchers think that being exposed to low-frequency electromagnetic fields (from common household appliances) may disrupt melatonin levels.

One study of postmenopausal women found that melatonin improved depression and anxiety. Studies of people with depression and panic disorder have shown low levels of melatonin. People who suffer winter blues or seasonal affective disorder (SAD) also have lower-than-normal melatonin levels. Melatonin causes a surge in the neurotransmitter serotonin, which may help explain why it is helpful in both sleep and depression. The benefit to taking melatonin as opposed to other sleep aids is that it is both safe and nonaddictive.

Melatonin is also involved in the production of female hormones and influences menstrual cycles. Researchers also consider melatonin levels to be involved in aging. Melatonin levels are highest when we are children and diminish with age. The lower levels of melatonin may help explain why older adults tend to get less sleep.

Melatonin is a strong antioxidant, and there is some evidence that it may help strengthen the immune system. It has also been shown to have powerful neuroprotective effects both as an antioxidant and in the prevention of plaque formation as observed in Alzheimer's disease.

The best approach for dosing melatonin is to begin with very low doses. In children, start with 0.3 mg a day and raise it slowly. In adults, start with 1 mg an hour before bedtime. You can increase it to 6 mg.

RESTFUL SLEEP

To support healthy sleep, which as we will see in the next chapter is critical to brain health and craving control, I have developed a special supplement called Restful Sleep. It contains a combination of nutrients designed to support a calm mind and promote a deep, relaxed, restful night's sleep. This supplement contains both an immediate-release and time-release dose of melatonin, the calming neurotransmitter GABA, a combination of the essential elements zinc and magnesium, and the herb valerian, which together may produce an overall sedative effect to help support sleep.

6

LEARN NINE SECRETS TO CONQUERING YOUR CRAVINGS

CONTROL YOUR APPETITE AND LIFE

When Stephanie got pregnant with twins at age thirty, she gained about 80 pounds during her pregnancy and never lost it. In fact, she continued to pack on the pounds as her twin boys grew up. With kids in the house, she kept the cupboards stocked with all kinds of chips, candy, and sodas. She initially bought these things for the boys, but then she got hooked on them too. She craved sodas in the morning for a quick energy jolt and craved salty chips in the afternoon, and she felt like she couldn't live without cookies and candy in the evenings while watching TV. By the time she turned forty-two, her weight ballooned to 270 pounds and her doctor diagnosed her with type 2 diabetes. That really scared her and she knew she had to do something *now* to change her behavior and lose some weight.

To jump-start her new lifestyle, she decided to go to a weeklong weight-loss retreat where they served calorie-controlled spa cuisine and offered dozens of fitness classes and activities. She did great while she was at the retreat. There were no sodas, candy, or chips in sight and no opportunities to eat anything other than what was served at mealtime. By the end of the week, she had lost several pounds, and her cravings had started to wane. Stephanie was very excited, thinking she was on the way to a new life and a new figure.

But when she got back home, reality hit. The kitchen was stocked with the cookies, chips, candy, and sodas she craved. Plus, after being gone for a week, the house was a complete mess, the laundry had piled up, and the twins' homework projects sat untouched, even though they were due the following day.

On her first day back, she jumped out of bed with the best intentions to eat right and go to the gym like she had at the retreat. She scrambled to get the boys ready for their early-morning soccer practice, and by the time she drove them there, she realized she had forgotten to eat breakfast. She didn't want to drink a sugary soda like she used to, but she needed some energy so she bought a diet soda from a nearby vending machine. When she got home, she was so hungry, she made a big bowl of cereal. She figured she would go grocery shopping for healthy foods later after she cleaned up the house.

About a half hour after eating the cereal, her energy dropped again, and she felt the sodas in the fridge calling her name. She tried to resist, but eventually the craving was too strong, and she gave in. Every time she headed through the kitchen to the laundry room to wash clothes, she thought about the chips in the cupboard. Then she figured that since she had already ruined her diet that day with the big bowl of cereal, she may as well have a few chips.

Then her husband told her they had been invited to a barbecue at the neighbor's house that afternoon and he had said yes to the invitation. Stephanie was really ticked off at that because she wanted to finish cleaning the house so she could go to the grocery store. At the neighbor's barbecue, there were chips and dip, tubs of ice-cold sodas, bowls of M&M's, and plates of freshly baked cookies on display.

GET SMART TO GET THINNER

"I saw your public television special and changed my eating habits completely. I feel like a new person! The best part? I no longer have the food cravings I once had. Thank you!"

—Kelly

Starving, Stephanie stationed herself next to the chips and dip and finished off the whole bowl before having a burger. After the burger, she told herself she wasn't going to have dessert and managed to resist until her husband brought over a plate of cookies for her. With them in her hands, she could smell the vanilla and chocolate and they proved too irresistible and she ate three cookies. When they got back home and Stephanie finally got to sit down and relax and watch TV, the boys ran into the living room with bags of jelly beans from the kitchen and ate them sitting next to her. She told them she didn't want any, but after a while she found herself mindlessly dipping her hand into the bag of jelly beans. So much for Stephanie's new healthy lifestyle.

What went wrong? Stephanie didn't want to be overweight, and she definitely didn't want to have type 2 diabetes. She had eaten well at the retreat so she knew she was capable of going without the snacks and sodas she craved. But at home there were so many temptations that she just couldn't control her cravings. Or could she? Was there anything Stephanie could have done differently to help her avoid falling into her old habits? You bet! Let's rewind Stephanie's day with a few tweaks to show how she could have gotten better control of her cravings.

At Stephanie's retreat, she learned a lot about the kinds of foods she should eat, and she knew that her kitchen wasn't filled with any of them. So the day before the retreat ended, she called her husband and asked him and the boys to throw out the junk food. She patiently explained that diabetes would take her life early and that he and the boys needed to help her, plus it would be good for everyone in the long run. Her husband agreed, as his weight had also ballooned and he had high cholesterol. She also asked him to pick up a few healthy groceries before she got home. When she got home and saw the messy house, she decided she would spend one hour a day cleaning up rather than trying to do it all in one day. But she was grateful her husband did as she asked with the junk food and made sure to give him a hug and tell him how much she loved him.

That first morning, she spent three minutes making a protein smoothie with the whey protein powder and frozen berries her husband had picked up for her. She took the smoothie with her and drank it while she drove the boys to soccer practice. She headed straight from soccer to the grocery store where she filled her basket with good foods. The smoothie gave her good energy so she didn't feel like she needed a soda.

At home, she put in her hour of cleaning and then fixed a lunch consisting of a spinach salad with salmon, blueberries, walnuts, avocado, and a little olive oil and lemon. Thanks to the good nutrition, she was able to think clearly during the afternoon. With the chips out of her house, she didn't feel them calling out to her.

When her husband told her about being invited to a barbecue, she decided to bring a few of the raw veggies she had bought earlier that day so she could munch on them instead of chips and dip. At the barbecue, she sat far away from the buffet table and asked her husband to bring her a barbecued chicken breast and a little green salad and *nothing else*. She asked him to eat any cookies as far away from her as possible so she wouldn't be tempted. That night, when the boys sat down next to her on the couch, they each had an apple. Stephanie made it through her first day at home without giving in to her cravings!

For many of us, like Stephanie, cravings can be the culprit that derails our good intentions to stick with a brain healthy program. But like Stephanie, you can make simple changes to your daily habits in order to get better control of your cravings. In this chapter I will give you nine secrets for conquering your cravings. First, I will help you understand how cravings can hijack your brain.

Why Am I a Slave to These Cravings?
Understanding the Brain's Reward System

You probably think that being a slave to your cravings is a sign of weakness. In reality, your cravings may be a sign that your brain's reward system has been hijacked. What is the brain's reward system? It is an intricate network of brain systems and neurotransmitters that are critical to human survival. It drives us to seek out the things we need to stay alive and carry on the human race.

For example, when we are hungry we are motivated to eat because food tastes good, and it eliminates hunger and cravings. Drinking water quenches our thirst and makes us feel cool and refreshed. It is the same with sex. The physical pleasure we feel from sex drives us to repeat the behavior. The brain's pleasure centers link to the emotional memory centers to create powerful memories that drive us to repeat rewarding behaviors. If we got no rewards from eating, drinking, or having sex, we wouldn't be motivated to do them and we certainly wouldn't last long on this planet.

GET SMART TO GET THINNER

"I always craved things like bacon cheeseburgers. But you can have burgers in a brain healthy way. Now I make them with extra lean ground turkey, avocado, and tomatoes, and I either use whole wheat buns or serve them in lettuce cups. They're delicious! I don't miss the beef at all."

—Roger

Many other things that are not necessarily crucial to our survival also activate the reward system, like listening to music, taking a warm bath, or looking at a beautiful painting. Then there are substances and behaviors that are actually detrimental to our health and well-being that cause the reward system to kick into high gear—cocaine; heroin; alcohol; gambling; and yes, even caramel fudge brownies, salty pretzels, and chronic overeating.

Let's take a closer look at the neurotransmitters and brain systems involved in the reward system so you can see how it works and how it gets out of whack. First, let's examine the role played by four neurotransmitters. Neurotransmitters act as the brain's chemical messengers, relaying information within the brain. The strength or weakness of each of these neurotransmitters plays an important role in your ability to stop overeating.

BRAIN CHEMICALS INVOLVED WITH CRAVINGS AND SELF-CONTROL

- Dopamine—Motivation, saliency, drive, stimulant
- Serotonin—Happy, anti-worry, calming
- GABA—Inhibitory, calms, relaxes
- Endorphins—Pleasure and pain-killing properties

Dopamine is a feel-good chemical. Whenever we do something enjoyable, it's like pressing a button in the brain to release a little bit of dopamine to make us feel pleasure. If we push these pleasure buttons too often or too strong, we reduce dopamine's effectiveness. Eventually, it takes more and more excitement and stimulation to feel anything at all. Cocaine, methamphetamines, alcohol, and nicotine all cause an increase in dopamine that make these substances highly desirable. The amount of dopamine released when drugs are taken is much higher than what your brain produces for natural rewards.

Drugs and alcohol aren't the only substances that can hijack your brain. As I have already mentioned, sugar lights up the brain's dopamine pathway similar to the way cocaine and heroin do. Let me tell you more about that fascinating 2007 study from French researchers. In this trial, rats were allowed to choose between plain water, water sweetened with saccharin, water sweetened with sucrose (table sugar), and cocaine. After just one day of sampling cocaine and the sweetened beverages, the rats overwhelmingly chose the sweet stuff. In fact, 94 percent of the animals preferred the sweetened beverages to the cocaine, which is considered to be one of the most addictive drugs available. Even rats that were already addicted to cocaine or that received higher doses of the drug continued to go for the sweet stuff instead. This led the researchers to conclude that sugar and saccharin can hijack the brain's reward system and lead to addiction.

The same thing can happen from eating too many high-fat, high-calorie foods like bacon, sausage, cheesecake, chocolate bars, frosting, and pound cake, according to a 2010 study from the Scripps Research Institute. For this fascinating trial, researchers fed rats a diet of either low-calorie chow or unlimited amounts of junk food. Not surprisingly, the rats that ate the junk food began to display compulsive eating habits and, after forty days, were obese.

What was intriguing is that the junk food diet effectively rewired their brain's pleasure centers. Just a few days of indulging on the junk food basically wore out their reward system and significantly reduced their brain's ability to experience pleasure. This means that they no longer got as much of a dopamine boost from the bacon and other fatty foods as they originally had, and they needed to consume more and more of it to get that same reward. Needing increasing amounts of a drug in order to feel the same amount of pleasure is one of the hallmarks of addiction.

And just like drug addicts who continue to use in spite of negative consequences like health problems, relationship troubles, and financial woes, the rats loved their junk food so much they were willing to withstand foot shocks to eat it. By contrast, rats that had been eating the low-calorie chow quickly stopped eating the high-calorie fare when shocked.

Also disturbing about this study is the fact that the changes in the brain's reward system appeared to remain for weeks after the trial had ended. When the addicted, obese rats were put back on their usual low-calorie chow diet, they simply refused to eat. They preferred to starve themselves than eat the nutritious, but boring, chow.

The link between sugar and addiction can do more than just make you overeat. Did you know that bingeing on sugar has been found to raise the risk for indulging in drugs or alcohol? Because alcohol is metabolized in the body the same way sugar is, eating sugar can fuel alcohol cravings, and drinking alcohol can trigger sugar cravings. Sugar addiction is common in alcoholics and often develops when alcoholics try to quit drinking.

Professor Bart Hoebel and a team of researchers from Princeton University have been studying sugar addiction in rats for decades. In one of their trials, they found that when sugar-addicted rats were deprived of sucrose, they started drinking more alcohol than normal. Similarly, rats that consumed more alcohol increased intake of sugar.

As many of you know from personal experience, salt can also be an addictive substance. In 2006 a researcher from Turkey published a study called

"Salt Addiction: A Different Kind of Drug Addiction." In it he suggested that if you look at the current method of diagnosing substance abuse, it would apply to many people who have salt cravings. Some of the criteria used to diagnose substance abuse include withdrawal symptoms (some people experience slight nausea when they go without salt), unsuccessful efforts to cut down usage, and use despite consequences (high salt intake is associated with hypertension and increases the risk for stroke and cardiovascular disease). That sounds like addiction to me.

One of our weight-loss participants is very familiar with the lure of salt. He used to put salt on everything he ate, even on watermelon. He had been using so much salt for so many years that he couldn't taste his food anymore. We told him to cut out salt, and after about three weeks his taste buds started to perk up and he could actually enjoy some of the flavors of his food. He told me that he went to a restaurant where he had eaten many times before. This time he was amazed to discover how delicious the food was. He realized he had never actually tasted the food before. He had no idea what he was missing. Limit your salt intake, or it can hijack your brain.

For anyone who has grappled with cravings for foods that make you fat and miserable, the notion that you can be addicted to certain foods may not come as a shock. The concept is simple. When we eat brain healthy foods, such as a bowl of fresh berries, our brains release small amounts of dopamine, which makes us feel good. When we eat things like caramel fudge brownies or double cheeseburgers, our brains pump out lots of dopamine, which makes us feel really good. This increases the saliency, or the relative importance, of caramel fudge brownies and double cheeseburgers in our minds. Soon we no longer get much pleasure from eating berries and begin craving caramel fudge brownies and double cheeseburgers instead.

GET SMART TO GET THINNER

"I've tried eating lots of diet bars, diet cookies, and diet candy, but I still had cravings. A lot of those 'diet' snacks have enriched flour, which is just like eating sugar. The effect on the brain when you eat sugar or enriched flour is the brain asks for more. I've found that the less sugar and flour I eat, the better."

—Janine

Exercise and green tea have been shown to be natural ways to increase dopamine in the brain.

Serotonin is thought of as the happy, anti-worry, flexibility chemical. Many of the current antidepressants work on this neurotransmitter. When serotonin levels are low, people tend to be worried, rigid, inflexible, oppositional and argumentative, and suffer with anxiety, depression, obsessive thinking, or compulsive behaviors. One patient described her thinking with low levels of serotonin like a little mouse that is on an exercise wheel and cannot get off. Their thoughts tend to go over and over and over. Serotonin is raised in the brain by its amino acid precursor, L-tryptophan or 5-HTP. Amino acids are proteins. Unfortunately, L-tryptophan does not compete well against the other proteins to get into the brain. Exercise increases L-tryptophan in the brain because the other proteins go into the muscles thereby decreasing the competition for L-tryptophan to get into the brain. Simple carbohydrates increase L-tryptophan in the brain, which is why some people can get hooked on cookies, bread, potatoes, and sugar as a way to boost their mood. Exercise and 5-HTP or L-trytophan are natural ways to boost serotonin.

GABA, or gamma-aminobutyric acid, is an inhibitory neurotransmitter that calms or helps to relax the brain. If you have suffered an emotional trauma or you are under a lot of stress, GABA may be depleted and your emotional or limbic brain may become excessively active, making you feel anxious, uptight, or sad. This can make you eat in an attempt to calm your limbic brain.

The amino acid supplement GABA can help, as can vitamin B_6, magnesium, lemon balm, kava kava, and valerian.

Endorphins are the brain's own natural pleasure and pain-killing chemicals. They are the body's own natural morphine or heroin-like substances. These substances are heavily involved in addiction and the loss of control. Cocoa and DL-phenylalanine have been shown to increase endorphin production in the brain.

Now let's take a look at the brain systems that drive you to seek out rewarding behavior and that regulate your self-control.

BRAIN SYSTEMS INVOLVED WITH CRAVINGS AND SELF-CONTROL
- Nucleus accumbens (basal ganglia)—Pleasure and motivation center
- Deep limbic system—Emotional memory centers, triggers of behavior
- Prefrontal cortex—Focus, judgment, and impulse control

NUCLEUS ACCUMBENS

Located deep within the brain in an area called the basal ganglia, the nucleus accumbens is the pleasure and motivation center of the brain. It is one of the primary drivers that trigger your behavior. Be careful not to overstimulate the nucleus accumbens or it gets sensitized and needs more and more stimulation to feel anything at all.

DEEP LIMBIC SYSTEM

The deep limbic system houses your brain's emotional memory centers and can drive you to action. According to my friend, addiction specialist Mark Laaser, Ph.D., your arousal template, the emotional basis for what turns you on and what sets people up for addictions, is likely found in the brain's emotional memory centers. Understanding your early life triggers for later life addictions is important in the healing process. My grandfather, being both a candy maker and someone I deeply loved, was clearly involved with my sugar addiction. For you, it is important to understand where you were and how old you were when you experienced your first pleasurable or arousing experience connected to your addiction. These intense emotionally pleasurable experiences often strengthen the neural tracts for later addictions, even if the experience happened as early as age two or three. The first experience gets locked into the brain, and when you get older you seek to repeat the experience because it was the way you had the initial arousal or pleasurable experience, like the first time you tasted ice cream, had sex, or fell in love. Understanding the triggers for emotional eating can be very helpful to breaking addictions.

PREFRONTAL CORTEX

The prefrontal cortex (PFC) is involved in impulse control, judgment, focus, and follow-through. It is the brain's brake, which reins in your actions and makes you stop and think before doing something you might regret. The PFC is larger in human beings than in any other animal by far. It is the part of the brain that makes us human. It represents 30 percent of the human brain. Compare that with 11 percent of a chimpanzee's brain, 7 percent of a dog's brain, and 3 percent of a cat's brain. Cats have little forethought and impulse control. The strength or weakness of this brain system determines in large part whether you can say no to temptations or give in to your cravings.

Why Can't I Just Say No? The Brain's Self-Control Circuit

The brain systems that drive you to seek out things that bring you pleasure and the PFC, which puts on the brakes when you are about to engage in risky behavior, work in concert to create your self-control circuit. In a healthy self-control circuit (see Figure 6.1 on the next page), an effective PFC provides impulse control and good judgment while the deep limbic system offers an adequate dose of motivation so you can plan and follow through on your goals. Healthy dopamine levels drive you to pursue your passions while a healthy PFC acts as the reins or the brake so you do not get out of control. When these chemicals and brain areas are in balance, you can be focused, goal-oriented, and have control over your cravings. You can say no to cheesy lasagna, pizza, and hot fudge sundaes.

In the addicted brain, the PFC is diminished and the drive circuits take control. When the PFC is underactive (see Figure 6.2 on the next page), it can create an imbalance with the reward system and cause you to lose control over your behavior. When this is the case you are more likely to fall victim to your cravings. Having low activity in the PFC often results in a tendency for impulse-control problems and poor internal supervision.

Researchers have been studying addicted drive circuits in the brains of substance abusers for many years. Thanks to brain imaging, they are now seeing similar brain patterns in people who have problems with gambling, sex, and overeating. For example, researchers at Brookhaven National Laboratory have been using PET brain imaging to conduct a series of studies on the inner workings of the brain's self-control circuit in obese patients. The scans reveal the same patterns of brain dysfunction found in people addicted to cocaine or alcohol, with lower dopamine levels in the basal ganglia. Other PET studies from this same team show a correlation between a higher body mass index (BMI) and decreased activity in the PFC, which means overweight and obese people are likely to have less self-control.

Anything that decreases activity to the brain robs you of good judgment and makes you more likely to give in to your cravings. Pushing on your brain's pleasure buttons too hard or too often can cause the brain's brakes to fail by decreasing activity in the PFC. Poor sleep, ADD, and head injuries are also associated with reduced PFC activity. Many people don't even realize they have had a head injury that has affected their self-control.

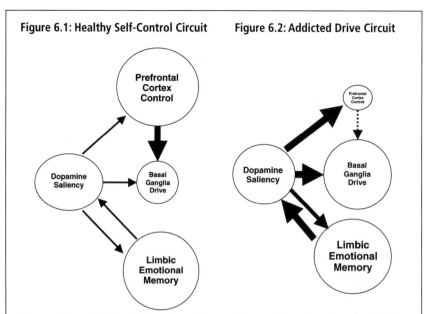

Figures 6.1 and 6.2: In the healthy self-control circuit, the prefrontal cortex (PFC) is strong and there is good balance between the chemical dopamine and the basal ganglia (BG), which houses the nucleus accumbens, and limbic or emotional circuits in the brain. In the addicted circuit, the PFC is weak, so it has little control over unbridled passions that drive behaviors. Addiction and chronic overeating can actually change the brain in a negative way making it harder to apply the brakes to harmful behaviors. In the healthy brain, the PFC is constantly assessing the value of incoming information and the appropriateness of the planned response, applying the brakes or inhibitory control as needed. In the addicted brain, this control circuit becomes impaired through drug abuse, ADD, sleep deprivation, a brain injury, or overeating, losing much of its inhibitory power over the circuits that drive response to stimuli deemed salient.

The Amen Solution All-Stars: Dr. Rizwan Malik

While I was writing this book, I received an unexpected e-mail from Dr. Riz Malik, one of the psychiatrists in our Reston, Virginia, clinic. Riz is an outstanding child psychiatrist who works very hard and has many grateful patients. The subject line read: "A Different Person." In the e-mail, Riz sent me the two photos you see on page 170 with a note saying, "Hey guys, I lost 28 pounds in the last three months. The pictures show the difference. I just wanted to share."

I was so excited to see the change in Riz, I had to find out how he did it. He said it was right around the time my book *Change Your Brain, Change Your Body* was released that a friend of his got diagnosed with high

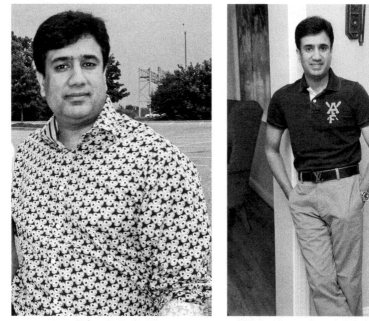

Before, 183 pounds   Four months later, lost 33 pounds

cholesterol and high blood pressure, and it scared him. It made him start to examine his own health and well-being.

After Riz came to the United States fifteen years ago at age twenty-five, he picked up the habit of eating lots of rich food loaded with saturated fat and drinking sugary beverages. He averaged about four sodas (about 400 calories) and two fast-food meals (about 700 calories each) during the workday, bringing him to about 1,800 calories *before* he ate dinner. For lunch, he was addicted to eating a burger with mushrooms and Swiss cheese. He craved them every day. He also craved Indian foods with heavy curry sauces and lots of bread to go with them (and the bread was made with white flour, not whole wheat). In addition, he also started to crave potato bread and was eating three to four slices a day with butter.

Riz said, "It seemed that eating all of this food was a way of rewarding myself for the hard work, the night calls, and the fact that I sometimes got overwhelmed with challenging psychiatric patients, as I had to 'absorb' all the negativity, sadness, and mental turmoil my patients go through. So eating was a good way out. But now I feel that I was, in fact, penalizing myself by eating all those carb- and fat-loaded meals."

Those high-fat meals weren't doing him any favors. In addition to pushing his weight to 183 and his BMI to 27, they gave him gastroesophageal reflux disease (GERD), also known as acid reflux. At forty years of age now, he thought that if he kept going in this direction, he would weight about 250 pounds by the time he turned fifty-five.

"When I started looking at what I had done to myself, I thought, 'My God, this is not good,'" Riz exclaimed. "I'm a physician and child psychiatrist, and here I am telling my patients and kids to eliminate sugar and eat healthy, but what am I doing?"

Riz realized he wasn't eating any vegetables or getting much fiber in his diet. Using the tips in *Change Your Brain, Change Your Body* as well as other reputable nutrition sources, he started making changes to his eating habits. He ditched the sodas and switched to water with a little lemon. He started eating organic apples and blueberries, yogurt with fiber, skinless chicken and turkey breast, low-calorie whole grain bread, high-fiber lentils, and lots of veggies. He also started taking fish oil and Attention Support, which supports attention and focus, and doing about ten to fifteen minutes of light exercise every day.

At first, the thought of giving up his burgers and comfort foods seemed almost impossible. "I thought, 'I don't like these healthy foods. I need some burgers and meat,'" he said. "But after a while, you get used to the healthy food and start to like it." Now he looks forward to his blueberries, yogurt, and other brain healthy fare.

After four months, Riz lost 33 pounds, dropped his BMI to 22.7, and whittled his waistline from 36 inches to 30 inches. He weighs 150 pounds now, but weight loss isn't the only benefit from the changes he has made. "One of the most amazing things is my sleep has improved," he said. "I had GERD, and now that's gone. Plus, my level of alertness is better, and I'm more efficient at work."

Nine Ways to Conquer Your Cravings

Now that you have a better understanding of the way foods and overeating can hijack your brain, here are nine strategies to help you get control of your cravings.

1. KEEP YOUR BLOOD SUGAR BALANCED.

Low blood sugar levels are associated with lower overall brain activity, including lower activity in the PFC, the brain's brake. Low brain activity here means more cravings and more bad decisions. In a 2007 article, Matthew

Gailliot and Roy Baumeister detailed the connection between blood sugar levels and self-control. They write that self-control failures are more likely to occur when blood sugar is low. Low blood sugar levels can make you feel hungry, irritable, or anxious—all of which make you more likely to make poor choices.

What causes low blood sugar levels? Many everyday behaviors can cause dips in blood sugar levels, including drinking alcohol, skipping meals, and consuming sugary snacks or beverages. High-sugar treats and drinks actually cause an initial spike in blood sugar, but then a crash about thirty minutes later. Gailliot and Baumeister's study also indicates that the body uses glucose less efficiently as the day progresses, leading to more self-control failures in the evening and later at night. This doesn't surprise me. I have worked with so many people who tell me they follow their brain healthy eating plan all day long but when nighttime rolls around, they can't resist the foods that tempt them. Does that sound familiar to you?

Here are tips to keep your blood sugar levels even throughout the day so you can reduce cravings and boost your self-control.

Consider taking the supplements alpha-lipoic acid and chromium. They both have very good scientific evidence that they help balance blood sugar levels and can help with cravings. (For more on these supplements and how they work, see chapter 5.)

GET SMART TO GET THINNER

"I used to go a really long time without eating because I was really busy during the day, but then I would be starving at night and have really intense cravings."

—Marty

Eat a nutritious breakfast every day. A lot of people skip breakfast. I used to be one of them. Don't think that skipping breakfast will save you calories and help you lose weight. In reality, it makes your blood sugar levels drop and makes you so hungry by lunchtime that you tend to overeat. That was the problem for Dan, the All-Star you met in chapter 1. "I'd get up in the morning and would have coffee but no breakfast until 10 a.m.," he said. "It wouldn't faze me until I was starving to death, and then I would pound down a huge lunch and huge meals for the rest of the day."

Eating a nutrient-rich breakfast helps get your blood sugar off to a good start and can help keep it balanced for hours so you don't get hungry before lunchtime. Studies show that people who maintain weight loss eat a healthy breakfast. For All-Star Dan, eating something for breakfast has helped him curb the cravings for bread, potatoes, and steak that would sneak up on him later in the day.

Add a dash of cinnamon. This fragrant spice has been found to help regulate blood sugar levels in people with type 2 diabetes.

Have smaller meals throughout the day. Big meals send your blood sugar skyrocketing only to plummet later on. Eating smaller meals helps eliminate the blood sugar roller-coaster ride that can impact your emotions and increase your cravings.

Stay away from simple sugars and refined carbohydrates. Things like candy, potatoes, white bread, pretzels, sodas, sweetened fruit juices, and alcohol cause your blood sugar to spike and then drop, so you feel great for a short while and then you feel stupid and hungry. Be very careful with high-fat, high-sugar, high-calorie foods because they work on the morphine or heroin centers of the brain and can be addictive, as you saw earlier in this chapter.

GET SMART TO GET THINNER

"I think of the foods I used to crave like an itch, and getting my brain balanced got rid of the itches."

—Renée

In 1994, a study found that carbohydrate cravings in obese people can be a symptom of a condition called chronic hyperinsulinemia, also known as insulin resistance, in which there is too much insulin in the blood. The researchers reported that this condition fosters carbohydrate cravings, and they suggested that decreasing the frequency of high-carbohydrate meals could lead to weight loss in people with this condition.

The bottom line: Eliminate sugar and refined carbohydrates.

When I finally got this one idea through my own thick skull, it made a huge difference for me, and I was finally able to lose the extra pounds I had been trying to shed for three decades. I love living without cravings. But for years I fought the idea of giving up sweets like Rocky Road ice cream and candy.

I know that kicking the sugar habit isn't easy for many people—it is kicking a drug—and it certainly wasn't easy for me, but I found that when I substituted brain healthy fruit like blueberries, bananas, and apples, the cravings completely went away. Have you ever known someone to eat too many blueberries? For most people, it takes about two weeks of completely avoiding sugar for your cravings to go away.

2. DECREASE THE ARTIFICIAL SWEETENERS.

If you really want to decrease your cravings, you have to get rid of the artificial sweeteners in your diet. We think of these sweeteners as free, because they have no calories, but because they are up to six hundred times sweeter than sugar, they may activate the appetite centers of the brain, making you crave even more food and more sugar. A group of Australian scientists found that alcohol floods the bloodstream faster when it is mixed with beverages containing artificial sweeteners rather than sugar. Diet sodas are *not* the answer. The one natural no-calorie sweetener I like is called stevia.

3. MANAGE YOUR STRESS.

Another very important way to decrease your cravings is to get on a daily stress-management program. Anything stressful can trigger certain hormones that activate your cravings, making you believe that you *need* the mashed potatoes, macaroni and cheese, or ice cream. Chronic stress has been implicated in obesity, as well as addictions; anxiety and depressive disorders; Alzheimer's disease; heart disease; and a host of immune disorders, including cancer.

When stress hits, there are increased levels of adrenaline (leading to anxiety) and cortisol (leading to many ills) and decreased levels of the hormones DHEA and testosterone (leading to loss of muscle tissue, increased fat, and decreased libido). Chronic exposure to adrenaline causes our systems to be overloaded with too much stimulation and leads to obesity, anxiety and depression, and memory problems. Chronic exposure to cortisol can make you fat, miserable, and stupid. It has been associated with myriad problems that make us unhappy, such as increased appetite, sugar and fat cravings, and abdominal obesity.

Cortisol signals your body to hold onto its fat stores, leading to a high waist-to-hip ratio (WHR—the circumference of the waist in inches divided by that of the hips), which makes you look like an apple. A person's WHR is associated with perceived attractiveness. An optimal WHR is 0.8; anything above that puts a person at risk for the illnesses mentioned above associated with higher cortisol levels, and less sexy. A WHR ratio of 0.7 has been associated with the most attractive women, in part because it is a sign of health and potential fertility. As we age, our figures go from being an hourglass to a shot glass (especially if we are drinking too much alcohol or eating too much sugar).

Long-term exposure to high levels of cortisol has also been associated with low energy, poor concentration, elevated cholesterol levels, heart disease, and hypertension, as well as an increased risk for strokes, diabetes (reduced sensitivity to insulin), muscle wasting, osteoporosis, anxiety, depression, irregular menstrual periods, lowered libido, and decreased fertility. High cortisol levels decrease immune system function, shrinking the thymus gland and impairing white blood cell function (as much as 50 percent following a severe stress). Chronic stress dramatically increases the use of medical services and health care costs. Stress not only increases cortisol, it decreases key anabolic hormones, such as DHEA, growth hormone, and testosterone. This combination causes you to store fat, lose muscle, slow metabolic rate, and increase your appetite.

In the last decade there has been a clear association between chronic stress, high cortisol levels, and memory problems, causing shrinkage of cells in the hippocampus of the brain. In fact, people with Alzheimer's disease have higher cortisol levels than normal aging people.

Here are several brain healthy ways of dealing with stress that do *not* involve food.

Deep breathing. As part of the body's natural stress response, your breathing becomes more shallow. When you take shallow breaths, it reduces the amount of oxygen that reaches your brain cells, reducing overall brain function. The simple act of breathing also serves to eliminate waste products, such as carbon dioxide, from the body, and shallow breathing can lead to a buildup of carbon dioxide. When there is too much carbon dioxide in your system, it can cause stressful feelings of disorientation and panic, things that can lead to cravings.

Diaphragmatic breathing, using the big muscle between your chest and abdominal cavity called the diaphragm, is a relaxation technique that can reverse these effects. Taking deep breaths with your belly also relaxes your muscles, which relieves tension, and helps your brain function more efficiently, which improves your thinking and judgment.

Here's how you do it. As you inhale, let your belly expand. When you exhale, pull your belly in to push the air out of your lungs. This allows you to expel more air, which in turn, encourages you to inhale more deeply. Take ten minutes twice a day to breathe in this fashion and stressful feelings will start to calm down. I use this exercise with my own patients all the time.

DEEP-BREATHING EXERCISE

Practice this simple three-step exercise to learn diaphragmatic breathing. Do this for ten minutes twice a day. Within a week you will be much calmer.

1. Lie on your back and place a small book on your belly.
2. As you slowly inhale, make the book go up. Hold your breath at the top of the breath for two seconds.
3. When you exhale, make the book go down. Hold your breath at the bottom for two seconds.

STRESS-RELIEVING BREATHING STRATEGY

Whenever you feel stressed out, use the following diaphragmatic breathing technique.

- Take a deep breath.
- Hold it for two to three seconds.
- Slowly blow it out (take about six to eight seconds to exhale completely).
- Take another deep breath (as deep as you can).
- Hold it for two to three seconds.
- Blow it out slowly again.
- Do this about ten times, and odds are you will start to feel very relaxed.

Meditation and hypnosis are also wonderful stress-management practices that can help boost your brain so you can get control of your cravings. I will talk about these more in chapter 9.

There are many other healthy ways to lower your stress levels without running to the refrigerator. Here's a list that you can refer to when you feel overwhelmed.

- Pet your dog or cat.
- Take a warm bath.

- Learn to delegate. You don't have to do everything yourself, and it is okay to ask for help.

GET SMART TO GET THINNER

"I have some friends who did the gastric bypass, or LAP-BAND, surgery who are still chubby. It makes perfect sense if you are eating lots of high GI foods constantly, even if you are only eating three ounces at a time, you are still messing up your system."

—Angie

- Don't automatically say yes to every invitation, project, or activity. Say no to things that don't fit into your goals and desires.
- Listen to soothing music.
- Lavender has been shown to have calming, stress-relieving properties, so use lavender-scented oils, candles, sprays, lotion, or sachets.
- If you're stressed about an upcoming event or situation where you have to give a talk or meet new people, rehearse what you are going to say.
- Learn to laugh at yourself.

4. OUTSMART SNEAKY TRIGGERS.

To control your cravings you also have to outsmart the sneaky triggers that try to sabotage you nearly everywhere you go. No matter which foods you crave, there are environmental triggers all around. If cinnamon rolls are your weakness, going to the mall and smelling the scent of cinnamon wafting from the food court can ignite your brain's emotional memory centers and make you feel like you *have* to have one.

Basically, you can't go to the mall, the airport, or the ball game without seeing store after store and vendor after vendor advertising something that will fire up your cravings. For example, whenever I went to the movies, I used to immediately think about getting a *big* tub of popcorn with lots of butter along with licorice. But then I actually thought about the gobs of saturated fat, salt, and sugar that would be flooding my brain. Another trigger for me is going over to my mom's house on holidays—she makes the most amazing pizzas. I could easily eat eight slices but end up feeling stuffed and stupid.

To control your cravings, you have to control your triggers. Know the people, places, and things that fuel your cravings and plan ahead for your vulnerable times. For example, I take a snack with me when I go to the movies now so I am not tempted by the popcorn and licorice, and I eat a little something ahead of time before going over to my mom's house on holidays, so that my brain can choose to eat a slice or two of pizza without blowing the whole holiday season in one thirty-minute gorge.

5. FIND OUT ABOUT HIDDEN FOOD ALLERGIES.

Hidden food allergies and food sensitivities can trigger cravings. For example, did you know that if you have wheat gluten or milk allergies and you eat wheat or dairy products, it can reduce blood flow to the brain and decrease your judgment? That makes you more likely to give in to your cravings. In addition, many of the symptoms associated with food allergies, such as headaches, sleep problems, lack of concentration, and anxiety, can increase stress and cravings.

One of the things that might surprise you about hidden food allergies is that the foods you are allergic to are often the ones you crave the most. It seems counterintuitive, but it is true. So if you have a sensitivity to chocolate, that may be part of the explanation why you crave it. A sensitivity to gluten could make you crave bread, muffins, and other baked goods. I often order a delayed food allergy test called IgG (or immunoglobin G) on my patients. If you suspect food allergies ask your doctor to test you for it or try an elimination diet. Dr. Annibali, our chief psychiatrist in Reston, wrote up the following summary of elimination diets for our patients.

Follow an Elimination Diet. We are coming to understand that subtle but important food allergies may result in brain inflammation that contributes to many of the brain issues we see at Amen Clinics. These food allergies can be delayed, in the sense that bodily reactions to the food items may occur up to several days after consuming the item. Conventional medicine has tended to ignore these reactions to foods. However, we believe that these food issues create a metabolic disorder that can lead to many "mental" symptoms, including fatigue, brain fog, slowed thinking, irritability, agitation, aggression, anxiety, depression and bipolar conditions, ADD, learning disabilities, autism, schizophrenia, and even dementia.

To test the theory that food allergies are involved in your issues, follow an elimination diet—essentially a dairy-free, wheat gluten–free diet—for one to two months. Also, consume no sugars, food additives, preservatives, artificial flavorings, or colors. If you find that you feel better after one to two months on this diet, slowly reintroduce food items, one at a time, every three to four days, to determine whether the newly introduced food item triggers problems.

When you reintroduce a food to which you may be sensitive, eat them at least two to three times a day for three days to see if you notice a reaction (unless, of course, you notice a problem right away—then stop immediately). Symptoms can occur from a few minutes to seventy-two hours later. If you have a reaction, note the food and eliminate it for ninety days. This will give your immune system a chance to cool off and your gut a chance to heal. Reactions to foods to which you have allergies can include: brain fog, difficulty remembering, mood issues (anxiety, depression, and anger), nasal congestion, chest congestion, headaches, sleep problems, joint aches, muscle aches, pain, fatigue, skin changes, and changes in digestion and bowel functioning. A good reference for the elimination diet process is *A Fast, Easy Allergy Diet for Behavior and Activity Problems* by my friend Dr. Doris Rapp. You can download the diet at www.drrapp.com for $7.99. In addition, you may find details on dairy-free and gluten-free diets on the Internet at www.gfcfdiet.com and at www.gfmeals.com.

6. PRACTICE WILLPOWER TO RETRAIN YOUR BRAIN.

Willpower is like a muscle. You have to use it or lose it. Self-control is very important if you want to lose weight and gain control of your life, happiness, and even intelligence. How do self-control and intelligence go hand-in-hand? Research shows that preschoolers who know how to delay gratification achieve higher academic performance, cope better with stress and frustration, and have better social and cognitive skills as adolescents. You can thank celebrated psychology professor and researcher Walter Mischel and his famous "marshmallow experiment" for this insight.

Here's how the 1960s experiment worked. Mischel or one of his colleagues invited dozens of preschoolers into a laboratory room one at a time and had them sit down at a table. On the table was a marshmallow. The researcher told each child that they had two options. They could either eat the marshmallow right away, or they could wait for several minutes and then get two marshmallows. Some of the children couldn't wait and gobbled up the marshmallow. Others, however, used an array of tactics to keep from eating the treat—clapping their hands or turning their chair to face away from the marshmallow, for example. (You can find several reenactments of this landmark experiment at www.youtube.com—just search for "Marshmallow Test.")

Mischel then followed these youngsters for fourteen years and found that those who were able to delay gratification fared much better in life than those who ate the marshmallow. The "waiters" had higher self-esteem, were better at coping with stress and frustration, performed better academically, scored an average of 210 points higher on their SATs, and were more socially adept than the "gobblers."

GET SMART TO GET THINNER

"With cravings, you get stuck in your habits. You just have to get unstuck."

—Sam

In a follow-up study, Mischel reenacted the experiment. This time, he included adults in the process. The grown-ups used a variety of tactics to avoid eating the single marshmallow while the youngsters watched. Then when it was their turn to try to delay gratification, children who previously had eaten the lone marshmallow used the techniques they had just witnessed and successfully managed to wait it out and get the two marshmallows. In later follow-ups, these children performed at levels similar to those who had the natural ability to delay gratification.

What Mischel's fascinating work tells us is that children can learn techniques and strategies to delay gratification. If kids can do it, so can you! Learn the art of distraction. Singing a song, taking a brief walk, or meditating for a few moments can take your mind off foods you crave. Put your trigger foods out of sight so they aren't so tempting.

Most of us learn to develop self-control as children. When our parents say no to us when we ask if we can do things that aren't good for us—have a plate of cookies before dinner, ride on the back of a neighbor's motorcycle without a helmet, or grab the tail of a strange dog—we learn to say no to ourselves. But maybe your parents weren't around much, and you had free rein to do whatever you wanted so you never learned self-control. Or perhaps your parents had no self-control themselves, and you learned to give in to your desires by watching their behavior. Or perhaps your chronic overeating has robbed you of your ability to say no.

No matter what the reason is for your lack of willpower, you can strengthen it. To pump up your willpower, you need to practice it. Make it a habit to say no to the things that are not good for you and over time, you will find it easier to do.

Long-term potentiation (LTP) is a very important concept here. When nerve cell connections become strengthened, they are said to be potentiated. Whenever we learn something new, our brains make new connections. At first the connections are weak, which is why we do not remember new things unless we practice them over time. Practicing a behavior, such as saying no to the doughnuts, actually strengthens the willpower circuits in the brain. LTP occurs when nerve cell circuits are strengthened, practiced, and behaviors become almost automatic. Whenever you give in to your cravings, it weakens your willpower and makes it more likely that you will continue to give in. When you practice willpower, your brain will make it easier for you to say no.

7. GET MOVING.

In chapter 7 you will discover why exercise is so important for a better brain. Scientific research has found that physical activity can cut cravings whether you crave sugary snacks or things like cigarettes, alcohol, or drugs. One study of moderately heavy smokers who had abstained from smoking for fifteen hours showed that even when faced with smoking-related images that would typically trigger cravings, the smokers had less desire to light up after exercising.

A 2009 study in the journal *Appetite* showed that cravings for chocolate decreased following a fifteen-minute brisk walk. The urges diminished even when the study participants were given a chocolate bar to unwrap and handle. Instead of immediately giving in to your cravings or focusing on how much you want something, get moving if at all possible.

8. GET ADEQUATE SLEEP.

Have you ever noticed that after a night with almost no sleep, you wake up ravenously hungry and want to eat anything and everything in sight? That is because lack of sleep increases food cravings. An expanding body of scientific evidence has shown that the less sleep you get, the more cravings you have, the more calories you eat, the more belly fat you have, and the higher your BMI.

ARE YOU GETTING ENOUGH SLEEP?

Age Range	Average Sleep Requirements
1–3 years old	12–14 hours
3–5 years old	11–13 hours
5–12 years old	10–11 hours
13–19 years old	9 hours
Adults	7–8 hours
Seniors	7–8 hours

Sources: National Sleep Foundation, National Institute of Neurological Disorders and Stroke.

Here's what researchers from around the nation have discovered about sleep, cravings, and your weight.

According to a study from the University of Chicago, people who are sleep-deprived eat more simple carbohydrates than people who get adequate sleep. The researchers studied twelve healthy men in their twenties and found that when the men slept only four hours a night, they were more likely to choose candy, cookies, and cake over fruit, vegetables, or dairy products.

For this study, which appeared in the *Annals of Internal Medicine,* researchers also looked at two hormones—leptin and ghrelin—that are regulated by sleep and involved in appetite. Leptin and ghrelin work together to control feelings of hunger and satiety. Ghrelin levels rise to signal the brain that you are hungry, and leptin levels increase to tell your brain when you are full. The researchers measured the levels of leptin and ghrelin before the study, after two nights of only four hours of sleep, and after two nights of ten hours of sleep. After four hours of sleep, the ratio of ghrelin jumped 71 percent, compared with a night when the men slept for the longer period of time. This made the men feel hungrier and drove them to consume more simple carbohydrates.

GET SMART TO GET THINNER

"Pretty soon, when you get away from the sugar and refined carbs, then you start looking for healthy things to eat instead of thinking, 'I wish I had a Big Mac.' "

—Allan

In a study published in the *American Journal of Clinical Nutrition,* researchers had people sleep for five and a half hours for two weeks and then eight and a half hours for another two weeks at random. Then they measured how many snacks the subjects munched during their stays in the sleep laboratory. When the people slept only five and a half hours, they consumed an average of 221 more calories in high-carbohydrate snacks than when they got eight and a half hours of sleep.

This pattern is occurring in the real world too, not just in researchers' sleep labs. According to the 2009 Sleep in America Poll, people who are having trouble sleeping are almost twice as likely to chow down on sugary foods and simple carbs, such as potato chips, to help them make it through the day. They are also more inclined to skip breakfast or other meals, which puts your blood sugar levels on a roller-coaster ride that's bad for brain function and often leads to poor nutrition choices later in the day.

Sleeping less makes you eat more sugary junk foods rather than fruits, vegetables, and whole grains. It also makes you eat more calories overall. A study from researchers at Case Western University tracked the sleeping habits and weight fluctuations of 68,183 women for sixteen years. The women were broken down into three categories—those who slept seven hours a night, those who logged six hours of sleep, and those who got five hours or less of sleep. They found that the women who slept five hours or less gained the most weight over time and were the most likely to become obese. The women who slept only six hours a night were more likely to pack on extra weight than the women who got seven hours of shut-eye.

Dozens of other studies point to a connection between a lack of sleep and weight gain or obesity. For example, researchers at the University of Warwick reviewed data from more than twenty-eight thousand children and more than fifteen thousand adults and found that sleep deprivation almost doubles the risk of obesity for adults and children.

A Stanford University study found lower leptin levels and higher ghrelin levels in people who sleep less. The researchers examined a thousand people, measuring their sleep habits, their sleep on the night before the exam, and their leptin and ghrelin levels. They found that people who consistently slept five hours or less per night had on average 14.9 percent more ghrelin (which stimulates appetite) and 15.5 percent lower leptin (which tells your brain you are full) than people who slept eight hours a night. These studies show that when you don't get enough sleep, you feel hungrier and don't feel full regardless of how much you eat.

One of the reasons why lack of sleep makes you more likely to give in to cravings is that people who get fewer than seven hours of sleep a night have lower activity in the PFC. Remember, the PFC is the area of the brain that is involved in impulse control, planning, judgment, and follow-through. Decreased activity in the PFC can lead to greater impulsivity and more bad decisions.

So, if dodging sleep has been contributing to making you fat, can increasing the amount of sleep you get help you lose weight? Researchers at the National Institute of Diabetes and Digestive and Kidney Diseases are attempting to answer that question with a clinical trial that is currently under way as of the writing of this book. The study is recruiting 150 obese people who average fewer than six and a half hours of sleep a night and is following them for four years to see how getting more sleep affects their body composition, belly fat, and more.

In the meantime, editors at *Glamour* magazine decided to put this notion to the test with an unscientific—yet fascinating—study. They enlisted seven female readers and gave them one simple task: sleep at least seven and a half hours each night for ten weeks. In addition, they were instructed not to make any significant changes in their diets or exercise routines during the ten weeks. The results were amazing. All seven women lost weight, with the weight loss ranging from 6 pounds to an astonishing 15 pounds.

Lack of sleep not only plays a role in cravings and weight, but it also reduces overall brain function and can wreak havoc on your moods. In addition to reducing activity in the PFC, it also lowers activity in the temporal lobes, which are involved in learning, memory, and mood stability. This makes it harder to pay attention, solve problems, and remember important information, and it makes you more likely to make mistakes. Sleep-deprived people are definitely not smarter.

They are not happier, either. People who are tired from lack of sleep tend to feel irritable and cranky. In one study, 44 percent of American workers admitted that when they are sleep deprived, they are more likely to be in an unpleasant or unfriendly mood.

If you want to curb cravings, get thinner, smarter, and happier, you need to get adequate rest. Aim for seven to eight hours of sleep each night.

9. TAKE NATURAL SUPPLEMENTS FOR CRAVING CONTROL.

N-acetyl-cysteine (NAC), alpha-lipoic acid, chromium, DL-phenylalanine, and L-glutamine are five amazing natural supplements that can help take the edge off cravings. See chapter 5 for more information on how they work.

THE AMEN SOLUTION | 185

GET SMART TO GET THINNER

"If I catch myself getting a craving, I take the Craving Control supplement and within ten minutes, the craving is totally gone!"

—Trish

Dr. Daniel Amen's Nutraceutical Solutions: Craving Control. Given what I know about craving and nutritional supplements, I developed a special formula to help support craving control. You can learn more about it at www.amenclinics.com. As we have seen, the key to controlling your cravings is balancing your brain and maintaining healthy blood sugar levels. In support of this goal, Craving Control supports healthy blood sugar levels while providing antioxidants and brain healthy nutrients. The formulation includes glutamine to reduce cravings, chromium and alpha-lipoic acid to support stable blood sugar levels, and a brain-healthy chocolate designed to boost endorphins. In addition, the super-antioxidant NAC is added, which has been shown in clinical studies to reduce cravings in a number of different conditions.

REV YOUR METABOLISM

GET IN GEAR WITH
PHYSICAL AND MENTAL EXERCISES

While conducting our study on retired NFL players, I made a startling discovery. I had assumed that these world-class athletes who used to spend hours in the gym and on the field to achieve peak conditioning would have continued some form of athletic training for the rest of their lives. Wow, was I wrong! I was shocked to find out that after they retire from professional football, many former players stop doing any kind of exercise at all. In fact, many of the former players in our study had turned into obese couch potatoes. It seemed ironic for me to be giving advice about exercising to men who, in their prime, could have run circles around me and knew more about exercise physiology. But I found that I had to give many of them a crash course in how exercise boosts the brain in order to motivate them to get off the couch.

By contrast, I wasn't at all surprised to discover that most of the people in our non-NFL weight-loss groups weren't very active. After all, it is no secret that our society has shifted to a sedentary lifestyle where most of us spend our days sitting—working on computers, watching TV, and driving. The problem is that a lack of physical activity robs the brain of optimal function and is linked to obesity, higher rates of depression, a greater risk for cognitive impairment—and worse. Physical inactivity is the fourth most common preventable cause of death.

If you want to lose your belly, get smarter, and be happier, you have to get off your butt and move! Physical activity is one of the most important things you can do to burn calories, improve mood, and enhance brain function. In this chapter, I will show you what physical activity can do for your brain and body. Plus, you will learn the best kinds of exercise for your specific brain type.

GET SMART TO GET THINNER

"As part of my new brain healthy lifestyle, I decided to start swimming. I started out swimming just four laps of the pool. Then after a while, I was able to swim fourteen laps, and I thought, 'Hey I can do this!' Then somebody told me that sixty-four laps in this pool equals one mile, and that became my goal, and I did it!"

—Ashley

Moving your body is only half the exercise equation. To supercharge your brain, you need to combine physical exercise with mental exercise. This chapter will also reveal the best mental gymnastics to help get your brain and body in gear.

Get Moving to Get Thinner

There is no shortage of research on the effects of exercise on fat loss. Decades of scientific evidence has found that exercise, when combined with a healthy eating plan, can help you lose the blubber and keep it off. Of course, exercise burns calories, which is one of the keys to weight loss and a trimmer figure. But burning calories isn't the only way that exercise can help you trim your waist. Check out these exercise benefits.

GET SMART TO GET THINNER

"I used to exercise for my butt. Now I exercise for my brain."

—David

TURN OFF THE OBESITY GENE.

Exciting new research out of Sweden shows that exercise can deactivate the "obesity gene." Haven't heard of the obesity gene? Scientists have identified a gene variant, known in scientific circles as FTO rs9939609, that predisposes people to obesity. A person can have no copies, one copy, or two copies of the gene variant, and your likelihood of obesity increases with the number of copies you have. According to the Swedish study, having one copy of the gene variant is associated with a higher BMI, greater body fat percentage, and larger waist circumference compared with those with no copies of the gene. Having two copies of the gene variant is associated with even higher BMI, body fat, and waist size.

What is so exciting about this study, which analyzed data from 752 European adolescents, is that those who had the gene variant but got at least sixty minutes daily of moderate to vigorous activity were no more likely to be overweight than those who had no copies. So even if you are genetically loaded to have a weight problem, you can blunt the effects of your genetic makeup. Your genes are *not* your destiny.

IMPROVE HOW YOUR BRAIN USES SUGAR.

Exercise increases your brain's ability to regulate insulin and sugar. Maintaining blood sugar stability is critical. If you're insulin-sensitive and you exercise, your body can handle sugar and insulin much better and you'll get off that blood sugar roller coaster.

REDUCE CRAVINGS AND OVERCOME FOOD ADDICTION.

New research shows that exercise is helpful in the prevention and treatment of addiction, including food addiction. Physical activity actually reduces cravings for addictive foods like sugary sweets and high-calorie, high-fat fare. When you eliminate your cravings, it can cut out hundreds or even thousands of calories from your daily diet.

HANDLE STRESS BETTER.

Working out helps you manage stress by immediately lowering stress hormones, and it makes you more resistant to stress over time. Raising your heart rate through exercise also makes you a better stress handler because it raises beta-endorphins, the brain's own natural morphine. Increasing your ability to manage stress can keep you from polishing off a whole bag of chips when you are under a lot of pressure.

GET SMART TO GET THINNER

"At first, I thought I weighed too much to go to the gym, but this program encouraged me to give it a try. I started going and just doing a little bit, like using some light weights. But it got the habit started, and now I go regularly."

—James

EAT HEALTHIER FOODS.

A 2008 study found that being physically active makes you more inclined to choose foods that are good for you, seek out more social support, and manage stress more effectively. As you are learning in this book, all of these factors can help you rein in out-of-control eating so you can lose weight. Obviously, choosing brain healthy foods over junk food provides the foundation for lasting weight loss. Creating a solid support network to encourage your new brain healthy habits can help you stay on track. And as explained above, getting a handle on stress is one of the keys to staying on track.

GET MORE RESTFUL SLEEP.

Engaging in exercise on a routine basis normalizes melatonin production in the brain and improves sleeping habits. Getting better sleep improves brain function, helps you make better decisions about the foods you eat, and enhances your mood. Chronic lack of sleep nearly doubles your risk for obesity and is linked to depression and a sluggish brain.

Get Moving to Get Smarter

Physical exercise is a powerful brain booster. Here are some of the many ways that physical exercise benefits the brain so you can make better decisions about what and how much you eat.

INCREASE CIRCULATION.

Physical activity improves your heart's ability to pump blood throughout your body, which increases blood flow to your brain. As you have already learned in this book, better blood flow equals better overall brain function.

GROW MORE NEW BRAIN CELLS.

Exercise increases great stuff in your body called brain-derived neurotrophic factor (BDNF). BDNF is like an antiaging wonder drug that is involved with the growth of new brain cells. Think of BDNF as a sort of Miracle-Gro for your brain.

BDNF promotes learning and memory and makes your brain stronger. Specifically, exercise generates new brain cells in the temporal lobes (involved in memory) and the prefrontal cortex (PFC, involved in planning and judgment). Having a strong PFC and temporal lobes is critical for successful weight loss.

A better memory helps you remember to do the important things that will help you lose weight, for example, making an appointment with your physician to check your important health numbers, shopping for the foods that are the best for your brain, and taking the daily supplements that will benefit your brain type. Planning and judgment are vital because you need to plan meals and snacks in advance, and you need to make the best decisions throughout the day if you want to lose the love handles.

The increased production of BDNF you get from exercise is only temporary. The new brain cells survive for about four weeks then die off unless they are stimulated with mental exercise or social interaction. This means you have to exercise on a regular basis in order to benefit from a continual supply of new brain cells. It also explains why people who work out at the gym and then go to the library are smarter than people who only work out at the gym.

ENHANCE BRAINPOWER.

No matter how old you are, exercise increases your memory, your ability to think clearly, and your ability to plan. Decades of research have found that physical activity leads to better grades and higher test scores among students at all levels. It also boosts memory in young adults and improves frontal lobe function in older adults.

Getting your body moving also protects the short-term memory structures in the temporal lobes (hippocampus) from high-stress conditions. Stress causes the adrenal glands to produce excessive amounts of the hormone cortisol, which has been found to kill cells in the hippocampus and impair memory. In fact, people with Alzheimer's disease have higher cortisol levels than normal aging people.

WARD OFF MEMORY LOSS AND DEMENTIA.

Exercise helps prevent, delay, and reduce the cognitive impairment that comes with aging, dementia, and Alzheimer's disease. In 2010 alone, more than a dozen studies reported that physical exercise results in a reduction in cognitive dysfunction in older people. One of them came from a group of Canadian researchers who looked at physical activity over the course of the lifetime of 9,344 women. Specifically, they looked at the women's activity levels as teenagers, at age thirty, at age fifty, and in late life. Physical activity as a teenager was associated with the lowest incidence of cognitive impairment later in life, but physical activity at *any* age correlated to reduced risk. This study tells me that it is never too late to start an exercise program.

PROTECT AGAINST BRAIN INJURIES.

Exercise strengthens the brain and enhances its ability to fight back against the damaging effects of brain injuries. This is so critical because brain injuries—even mild ones—can take the PFC offline, which reduces self-control, weakens your ability to say no to cravings, and increases the need for immediate gratification as in "I must have that bacon cheeseburger *right this minute!*"

You don't have to lose consciousness to suffer from brain trauma. Even mild head injuries that do not typically show up on the structural brain imaging tests can seriously impact your life and increase your risk for overeating problems. That is because trauma can affect not only the brain's hardware, or physical health; but also its software, or how it functions. Head injuries can disrupt and alter neurochemical functioning, resulting in emotional and behavioral problems, including an increased risk for eating problems and substance abuse.

GET SMART TO GET THINNER

"Every day, I walk at least a couple of miles, and I'm doing some running too. I take the dogs out and go to the track and do a couple of miles. My next goal is running three miles."

—Chris

Each year, two million new brain injuries are reported, and millions more go unreported. Brain trauma is especially common among people with addictions of all kinds, including food addiction. At Sierra Tucson, a world-renowned treatment center for addictions and behavioral disorders, our brain imaging technology has been used since 2009. One of the most surprising things the brain scans have shown, according to Robert Johnson, M.D., the facility's medical director, is a much higher than expected incidence of mild traumatic brain injury among their patients.

Get Moving to Get Happier

Have you ever heard the term *runner's high*? Is it really possible to feel that good, just from exercise? You bet it is. Exercise can activate the same pathways in the brain as morphine and increases the release of endorphins, natural feel-good neurotransmitters. That makes exercise the closest thing to a happiness pill you will ever find.

BOOST YOUR MOOD.

Physical exercise stimulates neurotransmitter activity, specifically norepinephrine, dopamine, and serotonin, which elevates mood.

FIGHT DEPRESSION.

Type 4 Sad or Emotional Overeaters need to pay special attention to this. Exercise can be as effective as prescription medicine in treating depression. One of the reasons why exercise can be so useful is because BDNF, which I wrote about earlier in this chapter, not only grows new brain cells but is also instrumental in putting the brakes on depression.

The antidepressant benefits of exercise have been documented in medical literature. One study compared the benefits of exercise with those of the prescription antidepressant drug Zoloft. After twelve weeks, exercise proved equally effective as Zoloft in curbing depression. After ten months, exercise surpassed the effects of the drug. Minimizing symptoms of depression isn't the only way physical exercise outshone Zoloft.

GET SMART TO GET THINNER

"Even when I wake up and feel sluggish, I know that once I go to the gym, I will feel better."

—Marisa

Like all prescription medications for depression, Zoloft is associated with negative side effects, such as sexual dysfunction and lack of libido. Plus, taking Zoloft may ruin your ability to qualify for health insurance. Finally, popping a prescription pill doesn't help you learn any new skills. On the contrary, exercise improves your fitness, your shape, and your health, which also boosts self-esteem. It doesn't affect your insurability, and it allows you to gain new skills. If anyone in your family has feelings of depression, exercise can help.

I teach a course for people who suffer from depression, and one of the main things we cover is the importance of exercise in warding off this condition. I encourage all of these patients to start exercising and especially to engage in aerobic activity that gets the heart pumping. The results are truly amazing. Over time, many of these patients who have been taking antidepressant medication for years feel so much better that they are able to wean off the medicine.

Fighting depression is very important if you are overweight because depression and obesity go hand in hand. A 2010 review of the existing scientific literature on the subject involving seventeen studies and 204,507 participants showed a significant association between obesity and depression. The link appears to be stronger in women.

Research shows that people who are depressed are more likely to be overweight and experience a faster rise in BMI and waist size than people who are not depressed. On the flip side, weight problems also increase the risk for developing depression. Which came first, the depression or the weight problem, remains to be seen. But there is no doubt in my mind that getting depression under control can help you manage your weight, and losing the extra pounds can help alleviate depressive symptoms.

GET SMART TO GET THINNER

"Now that I'm more active, I really want to go surfing. I never would have tried that before."

—Max

EASE ANXIETY.

Listen up, Type 5 Anxious Overeaters! Although the research on the effects of exercise on anxiety isn't quite as voluminous as the evidence on exercise and depression, it shows that physical activity of just about any kind and at any intensity level can soothe anxiety. In particular, high-intensity activity has been shown to reduce the incidence of panic attacks.

Disclaimer: Always check with your doctor before beginning any exercise program.

Best Exercises for Your Brain

Aerobic exercise, coordination activities, and resistance training have all been found to benefit the brain and help you lose fat regardless of your brain type. Even walking at moderate intensity can help you keep weight off after you lose it. In a 2000 study, obese women were better able to maintain weight loss than women who did not increase their daily physical activity. Walking is a great place to start if you are new to a fitness program.

GET SMART TO GET THINNER

"I had been riding a stationary bike but wasn't really getting my heart rate up. Learning about bursts changed that. Now I go really hard for a short time then back to my regular pace."

—Stephanie

GET THE MOST OUT OF YOUR AEROBIC EXERCISE WITH BURST TRAINING.

If you want a higher calorie burner, a faster fat burner, a greater mood enhancer, and a better brain booster, try burst training. Also known as interval training, burst training involves sixty-second bursts at go-for-broke intensity followed by a few minutes of lower-intensity exertion. This is the type of workout I do, and it works. Scientific evidence says so. A 2006 study from researchers at the University of Guelph in Canada found that doing high-intensity burst training burns fat faster than continuous moderately intensive activities.

If you want to burn calories with bursts, do intense exercise, such as fast walking (walking as if you were late for an appointment), for thirty minutes at least four to five times a week. In addition, in each of these sessions, you are to do four one-minute bursts. These short bursts are essential to get the most out of your training. Short burst training helps raise endorphins, lift your mood, and make you feel more energized. They also burn more calories and fat than continuous moderate exercise. Here is a sample of a heart-pumping thirty-minute workout with bursts:

SAMPLE BURST TRAINING WORKOUT

3 minutes	Warm up
4 minutes	Fast walking (walk like you are late)
1 minute	Burst (run or walk as fast as you)
4 minutes	Fast walking
1 minute	Burst
4 minutes	Fast walking
1 minute	Burst
4 minutes	Fast walking
1 minutes	Burst
4 minutes	Fast walking
3 minutes	Cool down

If you can't devote an entire thirty minutes to an aerobic burst routine, don't throw in the towel. Research from Massachusetts General Hospital in Boston shows that just ten minutes of vigorous exercise can spark metabolic changes that promote fat burning, calorie burning, and better blood sugar control for at least an hour. For the 2010 trial, researchers looked at exercise-induced metabolic changes in people of varying fitness levels: people who became short of breath during exercise, healthy middle-aged individuals, and marathon runners.

All three groups benefited from ten minutes on a treadmill, but the fittest individuals got the biggest metabolic boost. This indicates that as you increase your fitness, your body will become more effective at burning fat and calories with exercise.

BOOST YOUR BRAIN WITH COORDINATION ACTIVITIES.

Doing coordination activities—like dancing, tennis, or table tennis (the world's best brain sport)—that incorporate aerobic activity and coordination moves are the best brain boosters for all types of overeaters. The aerobic activity spawns new brain cells while the coordination moves strengthen the connections between those new cells so your brain can recruit them for other purposes, such as thinking, learning, and remembering.

GET SMART TO GET THINNER

"Getting an exercise buddy made it more fun to work out. Plus I felt more of a responsibility to show up."

—Sasha

What I really like about aerobic coordination activities is that many of them also work as burst training sessions. For example, in tennis and table tennis, you give it your all during the point, and then you have a brief rest period before the next point begins. It is the same with dancing, where you dance to the song and then take a short break.

In general, I recommend that anybody trying to lose weight do some form of aerobic coordination activity at least four to five times a week for at least thirty minutes.

Have you typically avoided coordination activities because you have two left feet? This could be part of the reason why you have a hard time controlling yourself around food. That is because the cerebellum, which is the coordination center of the brain, is linked to the PFC, where judgment and decision making occur. If you aren't very coordinated, it may indicate that you are not very good at making good decisions either. This could make you more likely to continue eating even though you are full or to choose the cherry pie instead of the cherries. Increasing coordination exercises can activate the cerebellum, thereby improving your judgment so you can make better decisions.

STRENGTHEN YOUR BRAIN WITH STRENGTH TRAINING.

I also recommend adding resistance training to your workouts. Canadian researchers have found that resistance training plays a role in preventing cognitive decline. Plus, it builds muscle, which can rev your metabolism to help you burn more calories throughout the day. Extensive research shows that adding resistance training to a controlled-calorie nutrition program results in greater loss of body fat and more inches lost than diet alone.

For example, a 2010 study from researchers at the University of Rhode Island compared body composition changes between two groups of dieters. Both groups followed the Dietary Approaches to Stop Hypertension (DASH) diet, but one group did moderate-intensity resistance training while the other group did not. At the end of the ten-week trial, the group that participated in resistance training lost 9 pounds of body fat compared with less than half a pound for the diet-only group. Plus, the resistance training group's thighs got skinnier while the other group's thighs remained the same size.

CALM AND FOCUS YOUR MIND WITH MINDFUL ACTIVITIES.

Yoga, tai chi, and other mindful exercises have been found to reduce anxiety and depression and to increase focus. Although they don't offer the same BDNF-generating benefits as aerobic activity, these types of exercise can still boost your brain so you can improve your self-control and reduce emotional or anxious overeating.

Best Exercises for Your Specific Brain Type

Which exercises are best for your individual brain type? In addition to the general suggestions for all types above, see specific recommendations for your type below.

- **Type 1 Compulsive Overeaters** Aerobic exercise boosts serotonin in the brain to help you get unstuck when you can't stop thinking about pepperoni pizza, potato chips, or mint chip ice cream. Be sure to vary your workout each time. This will help you learn to be less rigid. When you get stuck on thoughts about food, get up and move! One study found that as little as five minutes of exercise could help curb cravings.

- **Type 2 Impulsive Overeaters** Aerobic exercise helps increase blood flow and dopamine in the brain to boost the PFC and improve impulse control. People with this type need *lots* of aerobic exercise. At least thirty minutes every day is best, but make sure it is in an activity you love. If you don't love it, you probably won't keep it up. Also try a form of yoga that includes meditation, which will sharpen your focus and strengthen your PFC so you can make better decisions and reduce impulsivity.

- **Type 3 Impulsive-Compulsive Overeaters** Do an aerobic coordination workout for at least thirty minutes every day. Choose three activities you love, and then vary them throughout the week. Adding meditative yoga classes can boost your PFC and your willpower.

- **Type 4 Sad or Emotional Overeaters** Try aerobic coordination activities that are social activities, like dancing. Or join a local tennis club or basketball team. The aerobic activity boosts blood flow and multiple neurotransmitters in the brain. The social bonding aspect of the activity can help calm the hyperactivity in the deep limbic system and enhance your mood.

• **Type 5 Anxious Overeaters** In addition to aerobic coordination workouts, try taking yoga or tai chi for relaxation. Relaxation exercises can soothe overactive basal ganglia to reduce anxiety.

Don't think you can just exercise fourteen weeks and then go back to your old couch-potato ways. Several studies have found that the brain benefits of exercise are only temporary. If you stop exercising, your cravings are likely to intensify and you run the risk of falling back into your old habits. Make exercise a lifelong habit, like brushing your teeth, to help you stick with your brain healthy ways for the rest of your life. Find out how many calories you can burn from your favorite activities in appendix F or on our website.

The Amen Solution All-Stars: Patrice

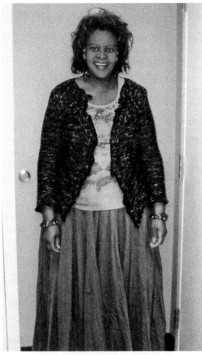 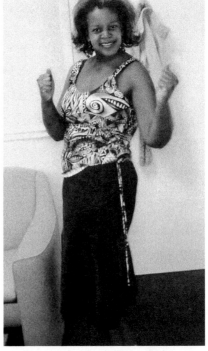

Before, 229 pounds   Five months later, lost 50 pounds

Weight had always been an issue for forty-five-year-old Patrice. By the time she reached the sixth grade, she already weighed 155 pounds. Granted, at 5'7", she was the tallest student in her class, but she was still carrying too much weight for her age. By her freshman year of college, the scale had already tipped over 200 pounds. Patrice often felt driven to eat regardless of whether or not she was actually hungry. She also found herself eating things she hadn't planned on eating.

Her previous attempts at dieting failed to change those eating patterns. Patrice had learned quite a bit of valuable information from a variety of other diet programs, but something was missing and she wasn't able to lose as much weight as she wanted to. All that changed when she joined the weight-loss group in our Reston clinic.

"Balancing my brain was the foundational missing piece," she said. "That was the miracle for me."

Getting diagnosed with adult ADD and getting the medication and supplements she needed to begin to balance her brain was the answer to her problem. It took a few weeks to fine-tune the right combination of medication and supplements, but by the fourth week in our weight-loss group, it clicked.

"For the first time in my adult life, my body didn't seem to be driven to eat when I wasn't hungry," she said.

Patrice still had to make dozens of good decisions throughout the day, but she found it so much easier to make the right decisions. After about six weeks, she realized, "I have new habits! I'm going to be able to do this for the rest of my life."

For Patrice, who was 229 pounds at her first weigh-in, the extra weight began melting away. After ten weeks, she had lost 22 pounds, but she didn't stop there. Five months into her new brain healthy lifestyle, she was down to 179½—under 200 pounds for the first time since college!

Some of the other keys to her success included counting her calories (something she admits she had never done before), weighing herself every morning, thoroughly completing the *Daily Journal*, recognizing and challenging her ANTs, and exercising, which she prefers to call "joyful movement."

Like most people who are Type 3 Impulsive-Compulsive Overeaters, she refuses to do any activity she finds boring. "You'll never find me on a treadmill," she said. But Patrice absolutely *loves* tennis, water aerobics, dancing, and group weight training at the gym, and she's hooked on the feel-good endorphin rush she gets from these activities. She also does yoga classes, which can help Type 2 Impulsive and Type 3 Impulsive-Compulsive Overeaters sharpen their focus, and strengthen their PFC to reduce impulsivity.

GET SMART TO GET THINNER

"I thought I was helping my brain by doing crossword puzzles every day, but then Dr. Amen said that just doing crossword puzzles is like going to the gym and doing right biceps curls and then leaving. I learned that I have to do a complete mental workout to have my best brain."

—Andrew

Pump Up Your Brainpower with Mental Exercise

The brain is like a muscle. The more you use it, the stronger it gets. New learning makes new connections in the brain, making you sharper and making your brain work more efficiently. No learning actually causes the brain to disconnect itself. Unlike a muscle, however, the brain gets easily bored and requires new and different challenges to maintain peak mental performance. Once the brain really learns something, such as how to play Led Zeppelin's "Stairway to Heaven" on guitar, how to knit a scarf, or how to swing a tennis racquet, it uses less and less energy to accomplish the task.

To keep the brain active, you need to give it a constant stream of new and different challenges. Acquiring new knowledge and new skills encourages brain health. Too many people, when they finish school, never think about the need to work out their brains.

I meet a lot of people who tell me they are keeping their brain young by doing crossword puzzles. I usually tell them that by doing crossword puzzles, they are working the language areas of their brain but nothing else. Just doing crossword puzzles is like going to the gym and doing right bicep curls and then leaving. A healthy brain workout is *not* simply doing crossword puzzles. You want to work out *many* parts of your brain.

Here are some workouts for specific brain areas that you might find useful. In general, I recommend that everyone, regardless of brain type, try to strengthen *all* areas of the brain. Building up certain areas may be more critical for you depending on your brain type.

- Prefrontal cortex (especially helpful for Type 2 Impulsive Overeaters and Type 3 Impulsive-Compulsive Overeaters)

    - Crossword puzzles and word games help the language areas of your brain.
    - Meditation boosts prefrontal function (more on this in chapter 9).
    - Hypnosis can help focus and boost prefrontal cortex function (more on this in chapter 9).

- Temporal lobes

    - Memory games
    - Naming games

- Basal ganglia (especially helpful for Type 5 Anxious Overeaters)

    - Deep relaxation
    - Hand-warming techniques (using mental imagery, such as imagining holding your hands in front of a fireplace or holding a cup of hot cocoa, to warm your hands)
    - Diaphragmatic breathing

- Deep limbic (especially helpful for Type 4 Sad or Emotional Overeaters)

    - Killing the ANTs (automatic negative thoughts)
    - Gratitude practice

- Parietal lobes

    - Juggling
    - Interior design

- Cerebellum (especially helpful for Type 2 Impulsive Overeaters and Type 3 Impulsive-Compulsive Overeaters)

    - Dancing
    - Table tennis (also works prefrontal cortex)
    - Martial arts, without risk for brain injury (also works prefrontal cortex and temporal lobes)
    - Handwriting
    - Calligraphy

Keeping up on the latest advances in brain science can also help your brain. Signing up for our free newsletter online at www.amenclinics.com can be good for your brain. My team and I give you the latest developments in brain science and how it applies to your life. When you read the newsletter, it stretches your neurons because you're storing more information and exercising the storage and memory parts of your brain. Good brain fitness, in other words, is more akin to cross-training at the gym—exercising in a variety of ways helps improve overall performance.

Here are three more simple ways to give your brain a workout.

BREAK YOUR ROUTINE.

This is especially important for anyone who is tethered to bad habits that are harming your brain and making you fat and unhappy. You can increase your chances of getting thinner, smarter, and happier if you change your daily habits and routines. Introducing new habits can help rewire your brain so you don't fall back into the same patterns of activity. For example, if you always take the same route home to work and stop at your favorite doughnut shop along the way, take a different route to work and bring a homemade brain healthy protein powder–and-fruit smoothie that you can sip along the way. Eventually, you will train your brain to look forward to this new habit rather than the old destructive one.

Here are a few ideas to get you started.

- For breakfast, make a fruit smoothie instead of having coffee and a cigarette.
- Make a new friend—someone who is living a brain healthy life.
- Contact an old friend you haven't talked to in a long while.
- Read a book about a subject that is completely new to you.
- Listen to a different genre of music than you usually do.

LEARN SOMETHING NEW.

Boost your brain by learning something new every day of your life. As little as fifteen minutes a day devoted to new learning can help optimize your brain. Here are a few examples of ways to spark better brain performance.

- Try out some new brain healthy recipes.
- Learn a foreign language.
- Take a class in something outside your major.

- Learn to play a musical instrument or a different instrument than you normally play.
- Try a sport you've never tried.
- Cross-train at work and learn how to do someone else's job.

SHARPEN YOUR SKILLS.

Although learning things that are completely new to you offer the biggest brain boost, taking your current skills to new levels by pushing yourself to improve is also beneficial. Look at the following for ideas on how to hone your skills.

- If you like to paint, try new painting techniques.
- If you play tennis, play against more-talented players.
- If you like crossword puzzles, tackle more-difficult ones.
- If you play guitar, try more-challenging songs.
- If you knit, try more-complicated patterns.

8

KILL THE ANTS

STOP THEM FROM STEALING YOUR HAPPINESS AND MEMORY, AND MAKING YOU FAT

Being overweight and being unhappy are not just eating or mood disorders; they are also "thinking disorders." ANTs stands for "automatic negative thoughts," the thoughts that come into your mind automatically and ruin your day. I think of these negative thoughts like ANTs at a picnic that infest your psyche and ruin your body. Here are some of the ANTs that have run through the minds of our overweight NFL players and weight-loss group participants.

> "I have no control over my eating."
> "I have to eat to comfort myself."
> "I don't like any of the foods that are healthy for me."
> "I'm fat because my family is fat."
> "I will never be successful at losing weight."
> "I cannot go out to dinner and not eat dessert."
> "I feel deprived."

GET SMART TO GET THINNER

"For a long time I thought I was too old to lose weight. That's an ANT."

—Nicole

If you have ever struggled to lose weight, you have probably had a few of these thoughts yourself. You may be surprised to discover that these ANTs could be a big part of what is making you fat, stealing your happiness, and reducing cognitive function. ANTs can attack anyone, regardless of age, gender, or brain type. Some types, such as Type 4 Sad or Emotional Overeaters and Type 5 Anxious Overeaters, are especially vulnerable to ANT infestations. Pay special attention to this chapter if you have one of these brain types.

When we talk about ANTs with our weight-loss groups and NFL players, the reaction is amazing. Many of them say it is the single most helpful thing they learn from our program. At our clinic in Reston, Virginia, where Dr. Lilly Somner leads the weight-loss program, the concept of ANTs resonated so strongly with the participants that it became the focal point of the ten-week program with several weeks devoted to ANT therapy. "ANT therapy was the one thing that made the biggest difference for people," said Dr. Somner. "They thought it was so important, they could have spent the entire ten weeks just on ANTs."

Learning to kill the ANTs by challenging your thoughts is critical to winning the battle of the bulge. In this chapter, you will learn how to develop an internal ANTeater to talk back to your negative thoughts so they won't send you racing to the kitchen cupboard or make you feel down in the dumps. Because getting control of your thinking is so important to your success, be sure to spend ample time completing the exercises in this chapter and make copies of them so you can use them whenever you experience an ANT infestation.

Your Thoughts Can Lie to You

Did you know that the ANTs listed above are *lies*? Most people don't know that their thoughts can lie. If you are overweight or unhappy, your thoughts probably lie a lot. Your thoughts tell you that you can't do it, you will never lose weight, you will always be fat, you are not good enough, you don't deserve to look and feel better, you will never find love looking the way you do, you will never get a promotion, and you are doomed to failure.

GET SMART TO GET THINNER

"Being honest with yourself and with others helps you lose weight."

—Rebecca

Are these lying thoughts helpful to you? No! They keep you trapped in your unhealthy habits. Australian researchers conducting a nationwide study found that the more severely obese a person is, the more likely he or she is to feel powerless to do anything about it. When you believe that you are powerless to change, you effectively give yourself permission to overeat. It is the little lies that you tell yourself, like "I have no control" or "It is my genetics," that make you fat and steal your memory and happiness.

That is exactly what happened to retired NFL player Big Ed White of the Minnesota Vikings and San Diego Chargers, who, at 365 pounds, told me that he had no control over his eating. I asked him, "Is that true? You really have *no* control over your eating?" He paused and said, "No. That really isn't true . . . I do have some control." But just by thinking that he was powerless over food, he gave himself the green light to eat anything and everything.

As I was writing this book, I was on a tour for my public television show *Change Your Brain, Change Your Body.* On these tours I often visit up to fifteen public television stations in two weeks. Even though they are a grind, I love visiting stations to help them raise money and support my shows. During a recent visit I was working with one of my favorite cohosts who was overweight. As we were talking at a break, she told me that she often went out to eat with her friends, always to places with "the unhealthiest food." She said it was her only social time and even though she wanted to lose weight, she was afraid of losing the social connections.

GET SMART TO GET THINNER

"I had no idea that my thinking had anything to do with my weight. It turned out it had a lot to do with it."

—Elsie

I asked her if she really thought it was true, that if she didn't eat at unhealthy places, she would have no friends. Sheepishly, she smiled. She had been watching my programs for years. "That is an ANT," she said. "If I believe that thought, then I am doomed to only eat at bad places. I am giving myself permission to die early."

With a simple question and a nudge, she got the concept. She did not have to believe every stupid, irrational thought that was keeping her trapped in unhealthy restaurants. If these ladies were really her friends, they could choose healthier places to socialize, or she needed a new group of friends. Are your friends' bad habits or negative thoughts killing you? I often say that ANTs are contagious.

How ANTs Can Make You Fat, Unhappy, and Stupid

Brain imaging shows us that negative thinking has a negative effect on brain function that sours your mood, slows your thinking process, and makes you more impulsive—*Pass the cheesecake please!* A study we conducted at the Amen Clinics clearly shows that negative thinking dramatically decreases activity in the cerebellum and temporal lobes.

Reduced activity in the cerebellum puts the brakes on your thought process and lowers impulse control. That is the last thing you need when the fast-food cashier asks if you would like to supersize your meal. Decreased activity in the temporal lobes is associated with mood problems, memory loss, and temper control problems. Talk about a recipe for weight gain! When you feel sad, can't remember the right things to eat, or fly off the handle, you are far more likely to reach for the chips and soda rather than the raw carrot sticks and green tea.

GET SMART TO GET THINNER

"Changing my thinking can help make me thinner? Wow, what a concept! Why hasn't anybody ever told me that before?"

—Brianna

Bad, mad, sad, hopeless, or helpless thoughts also release chemicals that make you feel bad. Your hands get cold, you start to sweat, your heart rate speeds up, you breathe faster and more shallowly, and your muscles tense up. These awful, miserable, negative thoughts can make you feel anxious, depressed, angry, or despondent. These feelings can take your PFC offline and make it harder to say no to your cravings.

In our weight-loss groups, the vast majority of the participants have absolutely no idea that their thoughts are controlling them and keeping them chained to their bad eating habits, dark moods, and constant worrying. When they grasp this new concept, they can't wait to learn how to kill those negative thoughts. Before I show you how to kill them, let's get better acquainted with various "species" of ANTs.

Ten ANTs That Are Expanding Your Waistline and Shrinking Your Happiness

Over the years therapists have identified ten "species" of ANTs or types of negative thoughts that keep you stuck in your bad habits.

1. All or nothing
2. Always thinking
3. Focusing on the negative
4. Thinking with your feelings
5. Guilt beating
6. Labeling
7. Fortune-telling
8. Mind reading
9. Blame
10. Denial

1. ALL OR NOTHING

One of the people I met on my public television show tour for *Change Your Brain, Change Your Body* said she hated the gym so much that she would never exercise. I asked her, "Do you like to dance?" And she replied, "Oh, I love to dance." "How about taking a walk on the beach?" I asked. "I like that too," she said. When I told her that dancing and walking on the beach are forms of exercise, she gave me a puzzled look. She had always equated "exercise" only with the gym. When she realized that any type of physical activity qualified as a type of exercise, she said, "Maybe I don't hate to exercise; maybe I just hate the gym." This is an example of all or nothing thinking, when you believe that everything is all good or all bad. Here are a few more examples.

"I haven't eaten any candy for seven days, I have got this licked."
"I just ate a doughnut. I am doomed to be the fattest person on the planet."
"We had an argument. I think it's over."
"I couldn't run a whole mile. I'm a terrible athlete and should just quit working out."

If you stick to your brain healthy eating plan for a month, you think you are the most disciplined person on the planet. If you stop for fast food one day because you didn't have time for breakfast and you're starving, you think you have no discipline, give up on your new eating habits, and go back to eating junk food on a daily basis.

Everybody runs into speed bumps and small failures in life, but that doesn't mean that *you* are a failure. A better approach is to acknowledge that you ate food that wasn't the best for your brain or your waistline and then get back on track immediately—not tomorrow. One slipup doesn't mean you should give up entirely.

GET SMART TO GET THINNER

"I didn't realize that by thinking, 'I'm never going to lose weight,' I was actually preventing myself from losing weight. Getting rid of that ANT helped me get rid of the weight."

—Eric

---

2. ALWAYS THINKING

This is when you overgeneralize a situation. Always thinking usually involves thoughts with words, such as *always, never, every time,* or *everyone.* Here are some examples:

> *"I will never be able to stop eating fried chicken."*
> *"I have always been fat; it will never change."*
> *"Every time I try to exercise, I get injured."*
> *"She's always in a bad mood."*
> *"No one ever listens to me."*
> *"Every time I get stressed, I have to eat something."*
> *"I don't like any of the foods that are good for me."*

Always thinking ANTs are very common. Beware when they creep into your mind, because they can have a very immediate, negative effect on your mood. Plus, they sentence you to a lifetime of overeating and other bad habits. Always thinking ANTs make you believe you have no control over your actions and behaviors and that you are incapable of changing them. When you find yourself barraged by an always thinking ANT, ask yourself if it is really true. For example, is it true that no one *ever* listens to you? *Ever?* Think of occasions when people have listened to you to help squash this pesky ANT.

3. FOCUSING ON THE NEGATIVE

So many people who are overweight and unhappy can find something negative to say about any situation no matter how positive it may seem to other people. This ANT can take a positive experience, relationship, or achievement and taint it with negativity. It is the judge, jury, and executioner of new experiences, new relationships, and new habits.

> *"I wanted to lose 30 pounds in ten weeks, but I have only lost 8 pounds. I'm a complete failure."*

GET SMART TO GET THINNER

"If you lose 10 pounds in ten weeks, that's good. But so many people want more than that and get frustrated. You have to change your mindset. Slow and steady is brain healthy, because you are learning new habits you can maintain long term."

—Riley

> *"I went to the gym and did a hard workout, but the guy on the bike next to me was talking the whole time, so I'm never going back there."*
>
> *"I started eating two servings of vegetables a day, but I should be eating five for optimal health, so I should just give up on eating them altogether."*

Focusing on the negative releases brain chemicals that make you feel bad, and that reduces brain activity in the area involved with self-control, judgment, and planning. This increases your chances for making bad choices like ordering a third 700-calorie margarita and eating a second bowlful of chips, or staying up so late updating your social networking page that you wake up exhausted and need to guzzle caffeine to get going. Focusing on the negative makes you more inclined to give up on your efforts to lead a brain healthy life and sets you up for failure.

GET SMART TO GET THINNER

"Now if I get on the scale and I haven't lost as much weight as I wanted to, I don't get down on myself the way I used to. I just stay focused on how far I've come already. It totally changes my attitude and helps me feel good about myself."

—Andrea

Try focusing on the positive, and it will improve your mood and make you feel better about yourself. Putting a positive spin on your thoughts leads to positive changes in your brain that make you happier and smarter and will help you stick with this program. For example, here's how you could think about these same situations.

> *"I have already lost 8 pounds and have changed my lifestyle so I will continue to lose weight until I reach my goal of losing 30 pounds."*
> *"After working out, I had a lot more energy for the rest of the day."*
> *"Eating two servings of vegetables a day is better than none."*

If you want your brain to work better, be grateful for the good things in your life. At the Amen Clinics, we performed a SPECT study, which found that practicing gratitude causes real changes in your brain that enhance brain function and make you feel better. Learning how to spin your negative thoughts into positive ones takes practice. Here are two exercises I recommend.

Gratitude Exercise #1

Write down five things you are grateful for every day. Use the form provided or use our online *Daily Journal* to write down the things you are grateful for. The act of writing helps to solidify them in your brain. In research from the University of Pennsylvania, doing a similar exercise boosted patients' level of happiness in just three weeks. This exercise is an integral part of our plan.

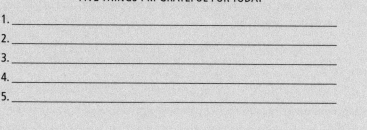

FIVE THINGS I'M GRATEFUL FOR TODAY

1. _____
2. _____
3. _____
4. _____
5. _____

Gratitude Exercise #2: The Glad Game

No matter what situation you are in, try to find something to be glad about. Think of a time when you were in a difficult or disappointing situation and started to think negatively but then found (or now can see) a "silver lining." Now try to explain the same situation from a "glad" standpoint. What did you find to be glad about the situation?

SOMETHING I'M GLAD ABOUT

_____

_____

_____

_____

_____

4. THINKING WITH YOUR FEELINGS

These ANTs occur when you have a feeling about something, and you assume it is correct so you never question it. Feelings are very complex and are often rooted in powerful memories from the past. Feelings can lie too. These thoughts usually begin with the words "I feel." For example:

"I feel stupid."
"I feel like a loser."
"I feel like nobody will ever love me."
"I feel hungry and must eat or I will get sick."

GET SMART TO GET THINNER

"When you walk around being grateful and noticing what you appreciate, you don't even have any ANTs."

—Jose

Whenever you have a strong negative feeling, check it out. Look for the evidence behind the feeling. Do you have real reasons to feel that way? Or are your feelings based on events or things from the past? If you feel like someone is mad at you, ask him!

5. GUILT BEATING

Guilt is generally not a helpful emotion. It often backfires and can be counterproductive to your goals. Thinking in terms of "should," "must," "ought to," and "have to" are typical with this ANT. Here are some examples.

"I should stop eating sugar."
"I have to count my calories."
"I ought to go to the gym more."

What happens when you say these kinds of things to yourself? Do they make you more inclined to cut the sugar, count calories, or hit the gym? I doubt it. It is human nature to push back when we feel like we "must" do something, even if it is something that will benefit us in the end. It is better to replace "guilt beatings" with phrases like "I want to do this," "It fits with my goals to do that," or "It would be helpful to do this." In the examples above, it would be beneficial to change the wording of these thoughts as follows.

"It is my goal to stop eating sugar because it will reduce my cravings, prevent energy crashes, diabetes, and inflammation in my body and get me off this energy and emotional roller coaster."
"I want to count my calories because it will help me learn to take control of my eating."
"It is in my best interest to go to the gym because exercising will burn calories and will make me feel better and more energized."

GET SMART TO GET THINNER

"I used to have ANTs running through my head all day long. Now I'm an expert ANT killer."

—Zoe

6. LABELING

Whenever you call yourself or someone else names or use negative terms to describe them, you have a labeling ANT in your brain. A lot of us do this on a regular basis. You may have said one of the following at some point in your life.

"He's a jerk."
"I'm lazy."
"I'm a loser."
"She's a slob."
"I'm a wimp."

The problem with negative labels is that they exercise negative pathways in the brain and make them stronger. Negative pathways can lead to negative behaviors, including the very behaviors you are trying to change. Calling yourself names takes away your control over your thoughts and actions. For example, if you are "lazy," then why bother trying to do some kind of physical activity? It is as if you have given up before you have even tried. This defeatist attitude keeps you stuck in your old ways.

Labeling others prevents you from seeing a situation clearly. When you call yourself or someone else a jerk, you lump them with all the other jerks you have ever known, and you can no longer deal with them as an individual or in a reasonable way.

Beware of the Red ANTs

These last four ANTs are the worst of the bunch. I call them the red ANTs because they can really sting and can prevent you from losing the muffin top, feeling happier, and getting smarter.

7. FORTUNE-TELLING

Do you tend to predict the worst? If so, you may have a fortune-telling ANT infestation. These ANTs can creep into anybody's mind, but they are especially common in Type 5 Anxious Overeaters.

"If I try to run, I know I will trip and sprain my ankle."
"I might be able to diet for a few months, but I can't change my habits forever."
"If I go to bed earlier, I'm just going to lie there awake for hours."

Predicting the worst in a situation causes an immediate rise in heart rate and breathing rate and can make you feel anxious. When you feel like this, it can trigger your cravings for sugar or refined carbs and make you feel like you need to eat to calm your anxiety.

GET SMART TO GET THINNER

"I live my life in constant gratitude now. That takes care of the ANT problem."

—Wendy

What makes fortune-telling ANTs even worse is that your mind is so powerful that it can make happen what you see. For example, when you are convinced that you will sprain your ankle, you run that thought through your head over and over and may actually imagine the physical pain of your ankle rolling even though you haven't even started running yet. This kind of negative thinking deactivates the cerebellum, which is involved in coordination and motor control. This effectively makes you more clumsy and more likely to sprain your ankle.

GET SMART TO GET THINNER

"I've been on diets that work for the first 10 to 20 pounds. I guess they are okay if you want to lose weight quickly and then gain it back. They are not a lifestyle change. I'm more impressed by the lifestyle change you get with the Amen Solution. It changes the way you think."

—Taylor

Similarly, if you are convinced that you won't get a good night's sleep or won't change your habits, you will be less likely to adopt the new brain healthy habits that could help you sleep better or shed those extra pounds. When you have fortune-telling ANTS, it keeps you stuck in your old ways.

8. MIND READING

When you think you know what others are thinking even though they have not told you, and you have not asked them, it is called mind reading. Mind reading is a common cause of trouble between people. It frequently happens in intimate relationships because one partner assumes they can read the other's mind. It doesn't work because you can never know what others are thinking. You are probably familiar with these mind-reading ANTs.

"He doesn't like me because I'm fat."
"They think I won't be able to keep up with them on our walk."
"They think I will never amount to much."

I have twenty-five years of education—mostly in how to diagnose, treat, and help people—and I can't read anyone's mind. I have no idea what they are thinking unless they tell me. A glance in your direction doesn't mean somebody is talking about you or mad at you. I tell people that a negative look from someone else may be nothing more than his being constipated! You just don't know. When there are things you don't understand, ask for clarification, and stay away from mind-reading ANTs. They are very infectious and cause trouble between people.

The Most Dangerous Red ANTs

Of all the ANTs, the blame and denial ANTs are the ones that hurt the most. Having these ANTs roaming around in your mind can prevent you from ever reaching your goals.

9. BLAME

Blaming others for your problems is toxic thinking. When you blame something or someone else for the problems in your life, you become a victim of circumstances, and you cannot do anything to change your situation. That keeps you fat and unhappy. Be honest with yourself and ask yourself if you have a tendency to say things like the following.

"It's your fault I'm out of shape because you won't exercise with me."
"It's not my fault I eat too much; my mom taught me to clean my plate."
"If restaurants didn't give such big servings, I wouldn't be so fat."

Whenever you begin a sentence with "It is your fault that I . . . ," it can ruin your life. These ANTs make you a victim. And when you are a victim, you are powerless to change your behavior. In order to break free from addiction, you have to change your thinking, so kill the blame ANTs, by making it your responsibility to change. It is your life. I love what Vernon Howard once wrote: "Permitting your life to be taken over by another person is like letting the waiter eat your dinner." It just makes no sense.

GET SMART TO GET THINNER

"I'm 5'4" and I weighed over 240 pounds, but I was in total denial. I kept telling myself that my weight was okay because I didn't have any major health problems like high blood pressure or diabetes. But it was *not* okay. I felt lousy, I wasn't happy, and I was getting mentally foggy."

—Toni

---

10. DENIAL

In the Australian study mentioned above, individuals with a BMI between 30 and 40, which is in the obese range, believed they could lose weight if they needed to, but they didn't feel it was necessary! Talk about denial! People who are overweight are often filled with denial ANTs. For example:

"I'm not as fat as my dad, so I'm still okay."
"I don't have diabetes, so my weight isn't a problem."
"If I get to 300 pounds then I'll start thinking about losing weight."
"I can stop drinking caffeine anytime I want. I just don't want to quit yet."
"I only binge when I'm stressed out, not every day."

Refusing to admit that you have a problem keeps you mired in your current state. If you don't believe you have a problem, then there is no reason to change your behavior. And if you don't change your behavior, you won't get thinner, happier, or smarter.

Kill the ANTs to Take Control of Your Thoughts, Moods, and Weight

Now that you are familiar with the various species of ANTs, it is time to learn how to kill the pesky thoughts. With the ANT-killing exercises in this chapter, you will discover how to turn your negative thinking into positive, accurate, healthy thinking. Did you know that happy, positive, hopeful, loving thoughts release chemicals that make you feel good? Scientific studies have found that changing your thinking can be as effective as antidepressant medications to treat anxiety and depression.

> **GET SMART TO GET THINNER**
>
> "My ANTs? They aren't here so much anymore now that I know how to talk back to them."
>
> —Ron

Take note, I am not recommending pie-in-the-sky happy, delusional thinking. What I want you to adopt is *honest* thinking. Honest thinking can help you feel happier, think more clearly, and keep you away from the buffet.

Strong scientific evidence shows that the ANT therapy you will learn in this chapter helps with weight loss. Researchers from Sweden found that the people who were trained to talk back to their negative thoughts lost 17 pounds in ten weeks and continued to lose weight over eighteen months, proving this technique works long term. And a 2010 study found that a twelve-week program designed to change thinking patterns helped binge eaters stop bingeing for at least one year.

Challenge Your Faulty Thinking With Your Very Own ANTeater

Develop an internal ANTeater that can kill all the negative thoughts that come into your head and mess up your life. Teach your ANTeater to talk back to the ANTs so you can free yourself from negative thinking patterns.

Whenever you feel sad, mad, nervous, obsessive, or out of control, write down the automatic thoughts that are going through your mind. The act of writing them down helps to get them out of your head. Identify the ANT species then talk back to them. Challenging negative thoughts takes away their power and gives you control over your thoughts, moods, and behaviors.

ANT-KILLING EXAMPLES		
ANT	Species of ANT	Kill the ANT
I'll never lose weight.	Always thinking	If I change my behavior and adopt brain healthy habits, I might be able to lose weight.
I'm going to weigh 400 pounds like my mom.	Fortune-telling	I don't know that. If I act now, I can avoid gaining that much weight.

ANT	Species of ANT	Kill the ANT
I'm a failure.	Labeling	I have failed at some things in my life, but I have also been successful at many things.
It's your fault I have these problems.	Blame	I need to look at my part of the problems and look for ways I can make the situation better.

My ANTeater Chart

Whenever you feel sad, mad, nervous, obsessive, or out of control, use the following chart to write out your thoughts and talk back to them. You can also find interactive ANT-killing exercises on our website.

Ant	Species	ANTeater
_____	_____	_____
_____	_____	_____
_____	_____	_____
_____	_____	_____

Do The Work

One of my favorite books, *Loving What Is,* comes from a close friend, Byron Katie. In this very wise book, Katie, as her friends call her, describes an amazing transformation that took place in her own life. At the age of forty-three, Katie, who had spent the previous ten years of her life in a downward spiral of rage, addiction, despair, and suicidal depression, woke up one morning on the floor of a halfway house to discover that all those horrible emotions were gone. In their place were feelings of utter joy and happiness.

Katie's great revelation, which came in 1986, was that it is not life that makes us feel depressed, angry, abandoned, and despairing. Rather, it is our *thoughts* that make us feel that way. This insight led Katie to the notion that our thoughts could just as easily make us feel happy, calm, connected, and joyful.

It also led her to realize that our minds and our thoughts affect our bodies. "The body is never our problem. Our problem is always a thought that we innocently believe," she wrote in her book *On Health, Sickness, and Death*. In the same book, she also wrote, "Bodies don't crave, bodies don't want, bodies don't know, don't care, don't get hungry or thirsty. It is what that mind attaches—ice cream, alcohol, drugs, sex, money—that the body reflects. There are no physical addictions, only mental ones. Body follows mind. It doesn't have a choice."

Katie also writes, "It's only when I believe a stressful thought that I get hurt. And I'm the one who's hurting me by believing what I think. This is very good news, because it means that I don't have to get someone else to stop hurting me. I'm the one who can stop hurting me. It's within my power."

GET SMART TO GET THINNER

"I used to get so stressed out every time I weighed myself. Now I just think of the number on the scale as information rather than getting emotional about it and letting it upset me."

—Brittany

Katie wanted to share her revelation with others to help them end their suffering by changing their thinking. She developed a simple method of inquiry called the Work to question our thoughts. The Work is simple and very effective, which is why I love it. It consists of writing down any bothersome, worrisome, or negative thoughts, then asking ourselves four questions, and then doing a turnaround.

1. *Is it true? (Is the negative thought true?)*
2. *Can I absolutely know that it is true?*
3. *How do I react when I think that thought?*
4. *Who would I be without the thought? Or how would I feel if I didn't have the thought?*

After you answer the four questions, you take your original thought and turn it around to its opposite and then ask yourself whether the opposite of the original thought is true. Then, turn the original thought around and apply it to yourself (how does the opposite of the thought apply to me personally?). Then, turn the thought around to the other person if the thought involves another person (how does the opposite apply to the other person?).

I have done the Work myself many, many times, and it helped me get through a very painful period of grief. When I did the Work, I immediately felt better. I was more relaxed, less anxious, and more honest in dealing with my own thoughts and emotions. Now I always carry the four questions with me, and I use them a lot in my practice and with my friends and family. Here

THE AMEN SOLUTION | 221

is an example of how to use the four questions to kill the ANTs that are keeping you in chains.

Example of the Work

Cindy, forty-eight, had been overeating since she was in college. She was obese for about three decades and had diabetes, high blood pressure, and high triglycerides. Her family and friends wanted her to lose weight so she could get healthy. Cindy desperately wanted to lose weight but didn't believe she could control her cravings. "I have no control over my cravings," she told me. Here is how she worked on that thought.

Negative Thought: "I have no control over my cravings."

Question #1: Is it true that you cannot control your cravings?

"Yes," she said.

Question #2: Can you absolutely know that it is true that you cannot control your cravings?

At first she said yes, she knew she couldn't do it because she had been giving in to her cravings for nearly thirty years. Then she thought about it and said, "Well, I have never tried the strategies you recommend for controlling cravings, so I cannot be sure." Take time and meditate on each of your answers.

Question #3: How do you feel when you have the thought "I cannot control my cravings"?

"I feel depressed, guilt ridden, hopeless, and shameful because I believe I will always be fat and will probably die early because of it. Believing this thought makes me want to eat more."

Question #4: Who would you be without the thought "I cannot control my cravings"?

Cindy took some time here because the notion was so foreign to her. After a while, she said, "I wouldn't feel so much like a failure. And if I didn't think I was a failure, I might be more willing to try to change."

Turnaround: What is the opposite thought of "I cannot control my cravings"? Is this thought true or truer than the original thought?

GET SMART TO GET THINNER

"It was not as hard as I thought to change my thinking habits, and it is a much healthier way to lose weight and keep it off."

—Lori

Cindy said the opposite thought is "I can control my cravings." She thought about this for a while and said that if she used all the craving control strategies in this book, it might be true. She still wasn't convinced, but this was beginning to open the door to a new way of thinking for Cindy.

Turnaround to the self: How can you turn the thought "I cannot control my cravings"? around to yourself?

Cindy thought about it and said, "My cravings cannot control me." As she uttered these words, it was as if a lightbulb turned on in her brain. She finally got it. She understood that by believing that she had no control over her cravings, she was giving her cravings the power to control her. Looking at her thoughts from a different perspective gave her the push she needed to do something about her weight.

The Work Exercise

Do the following Work Exercise (based on the teachings of my good friend Byron Katie) every day to investigate and turn around the negative thoughts and beliefs that fuel anxiety, depression, and overeating. Doing the Work helps you see the truth of your life so clearly that negative emotions and thoughts have no choice but to disappear. What a comfort! Important: You must complete at least seventy written exercises in order to rewire your brain so that you start seeing reality for what it is, instead of telling yourself lies. If you do the Work once a day, that means you need to do it for ten weeks to effectively retrain your brain and change your thinking patterns. You can also do interactive exercises using the Work on our website.

Write down the negative thought or belief: _____

_____

1. Is it true? (Close your eyes, be still, go deeply as you contemplate your answer. If your answer is no, continue to Question 3.)

     Yes _____   No _____

2. Can you absolutely know that it's true? (Can you know more than God/reality?)

     Yes _____   No _____

3. How do you feel when you have the thought (when you believe that thought)? (Pay attention to your body, mind, heart, and self-esteem.)

_____

_____

4. Who would you be without the thought? (How would you feel or live life differently if you didn't believe the thought?)

_____

_____

_____

Turn the thought around. (Statements can be turned around to yourself, to the other, to the opposite, and to "my thinking" wherever it applies. Find a minimum of three genuine examples in your life where each turnaround is as true or truer than your original statement.)

_____

_____

_____

The Amen Solution All-Stars: Carlos

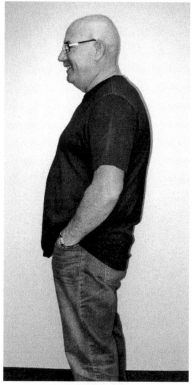

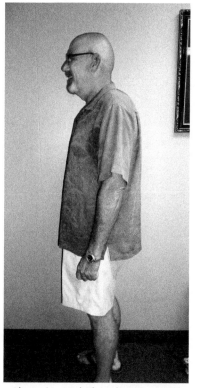

Before, 266 pounds

About six months later, lost 50 pounds

Carlos, forty-nine, knows a lot about ANTs. His mind was filled with worries and negative thoughts that sometimes sparked angry behavior. He had also experienced brain trauma due to a concussion and had problems with impulsivity. Whenever he saw food, he ate it. His diet consisted of whatever he wanted at that particular moment. Hash browns were a favorite.

When he joined our weight-loss group at 266 pounds, he learned that the foods he was eating were contributing to his ANT population. "I realized that eating crap just made me more hungry and left me feeling sluggish. Then the negative thoughts would come," he said. He also used food as a way to medicate his feelings of sadness and said, "I was always looking for something to make me happy."

By learning to kill the ANTs, he no longer eats to medicate his negative emotions. And by eating brain healthy foods, he has balanced his energy levels so he doesn't have those energy crashes that made him so vulnerable to ANTs. Carlos also started taking supplements, including fish oil and GABA, which he says took away the anxiety he felt. Conquering his ANTs helped him shed 24 pounds in ten weeks, and he is still losing—he's currently down 50 pounds since starting the program, bringing him down to 216 pounds.

9

PRACTICE DIRECTED FOCUS

HYPNOSIS AND MEDITATION

Jo-Ellen came to see me at age fifty for help with her weight. She had tried diet after diet and program after program with no success. At 5'4" and 200 pounds, she was 80 pounds overweight. She told me she thought she was highly hypnotizable because she had been hypnotized as part of a stage show in Las Vegas. She said she did everything the hypnotist suggested but did not remember a thing about it, just what her friends told her. Stage hypnotists are usually very good at picking out people who are highly hypnotizable to remain on stage for their shows. Even though medical hypnosis and stage hypnosis are worlds apart from their intentions, they do share some commonalities.

Jo-Ellen easily went into a hypnotic trance, relaxed deeply, and enjoyed the experience immensely. For the first three sessions, however, she did not notice any changes in her behavior. The fourth session was pivotal for her. In this session, I brought her back to when she first started to gain weight. She had been under stress in her first marriage after she found out her husband had cheated on her. She had two small children and felt trapped. She began to eat as a way to deal with her stress. Her husband would not go to marital therapy and continued his wandering ways. Even though she divorced him several years later, her pattern of dealing with stress through eating was set into place.

GET SMART TO GET THINNER

"It's one thing to tell people to watch what you eat and exercise. It's another thing to show you how to use your brain to help you follow through and change your lifestyle."

—Matt

After her marriage came to an end, she had several short-term relationships, but nothing that lasted. Food became her one true love. In the trance, I suggested to her that by overeating she was cheating on herself, cheating on her health, cheating on her children, and cheating on the people who would potentially be in a relationship with her. She could let go of her anger at her ex-husband and start doing a much better job at loving herself. Over the next few sessions, she began to do much better at letting go of anger and loving herself without overeating, and she started to lose the weight she wanted.

Of course, I also gave her fish oil, enhanced her vitamin D level, and did everything else in our program. She lost 80 pounds over the next year and was able to keep it off for the additional year we had contact. For many people, when you add hypnosis to a healthy weight-loss program, you can uncover the reasons for overeating and dramatically improve the outcomes. Hypnosis can also help people learn positive eating behaviors and create healthy long-term patterns of food intake.

Carissa, age forty-three, saw me for ADD, weight loss, depression, and alcohol abuse. Over time she did dramatically better, but weight still remained an issue for her. Under a hypnotic trance we discovered that she was fearful of getting thin because she had cheated on her first husband while intoxicated and hated herself so much that she never wanted to do that again. If she got thin, she imagined that she would be more likely to cheat on her new husband, whom she adored. Being overweight was her unconscious way of staying faithful. When we examined the misguided logic underlying her beliefs, she was able to lose the weight she wanted. She realized with a better body and brain, she would make better decisions overall.

Laura, thirty-six, came to see me for being overweight. She had struggled with her weight her whole adult life, but as a teenager she was thin. In a hypnotic trance we uncovered that she had been assaulted as a young woman and she unconsciously overate as a way to protect herself. When I helped her heal the trauma, it was much easier for her to lose weight. If you have suffered emotional trauma, then hypnosis, meditation, and psychotherapy can be very helpful.

In this chapter you will discover how to use hypnosis as well as other mindful techniques, including meditation, to help you lose the fat and boost your brain. I have personally been using hypnosis, meditation, and other techniques in my practice for many years and have seen these techniques help many patients in their weight-loss and mind-enhancement efforts.

Slim Your Hips with Hypnosis

To use hypnosis effectively for weight loss, it needs to be combined with a responsible weight-management program like the Amen Solution. Research dating back to the 1950s suggests that hypnosis can be a powerful, long-lasting weight-loss aid that can increase the amount of weight you lose over time. Here is a sampling of some of the most compelling evidence throughout the years:

- In 1959 in one of the earliest studies on hypnosis and weight loss, a researcher used group hypnosis to make dietary suggestions to study subjects. After four months, the average weight loss in the group was 27 pounds.

- In 1985 a trio of researchers analyzed the effect of adding hypnosis to a nine-week behavioral weight-loss program. The team divided 109 volunteers ages seventeen to sixty-seven into hypnosis and non-hypnosis groups. By the end of the nine weeks, both groups had lost a significant amount of weight. At the eight-month and two-year follow-ups, however, the non-hypnosis group had not lost any more weight whereas the hypnosis group had lost a significant amount of additional weight.

GET SMART TO GET THINNER

"I wasn't sure if hypnosis could help me stop eating sweets, but I find that since I was hypnotized, I think twice before automatically saying yes to dessert."

—Aman

- A study appearing in a 1986 issue of the *Journal of Consulting and Clinical Psychology* tested the effectiveness of hypnosis on weight loss in sixty women between the ages of twenty and sixty-five who were at least 20 percent overweight. The researchers divided the women into hypnosis and non-hypnosis groups and analyzed weight loss immediately at the end of the study period and again after a six-month follow-up. In the hypnosis group, the women received both group and individual hypnosis designed to enhance motivation, improve decision making, identify unconscious weight-related issues, and offer weight-loss suggestions. After one month, the non-hypnosis group lost 1½ pounds while the hypnosis group lost 8 pounds. At the six-month follow-up, the hypnosis group had dropped an average of 17 pounds whereas the non-hypnosis group had regained 1 pound, bringing their average weight loss to only half a pound.

- A 1996 review comparing weight-loss studies with and without hypnosis found that adding hypnosis significantly improved weight loss. The average posttreatment weight loss without hypnosis was 6.0 pounds; with hypnosis it was nearly double that at 11.83 pounds. This represents a 97 percent increase in weight loss. A further follow-up found the mean weight loss was 6.03 pounds without hypnosis and 14.88 pounds with hypnosis—that is nearly nine additional pounds lost thanks to hypnosis. This means the benefits of hypnosis increased over time, and people continued to lose weight long after the hypnotherapy sessions had ended.

- A pair of British scientists conducted a 2005 review of the scientific literature on complementary therapies (hypnotherapy, acupuncture, acupressure, diet pills, and homeopathy) used for weight loss. They concluded that hypnotherapy and diet pills were the only therapies that resulted in reductions in body weight, but they noted that diet pills came with certain risks. Hypnotherapy emerged as the only therapy that produced weight loss without any adverse consequences.

Let Hypnosis Help You Get Smarter and Happier Too

In addition to helping you lose weight, hypnosis can also help decrease irritable bowel syndrome, stress, anxiety, insomnia, pain, and negative thinking patterns. It has also been shown to aid in diabetes control and enhance mood. All of these conditions have a negative effect on overall brain function, make you feel bad, and increase the potential for overeating and weight gain. By addressing those issues through hypnosis, you can be a more positive, happy person. Recent brain imaging studies have shown that hypnosis boosts overall blood flow to the brain, which helps to keep the brain young.

Will Hypnosis Work for You?

Are you concerned that you might not be able to be hypnotized? Are you afraid that you might never "come to"? Do you worry that while hypnotized you might be forced to do something embarrassing? You're not alone. I hear these kinds of concerns from people all the time. Let me reassure you by answering some of the most common questions I hear.

WHAT IF I CAN'T BE HYPNOTIZED?

Eighty-five percent of people or more can be hypnotized to some degree if you can relax and follow some simple instructions. In my experience, I have found that most people who want to be hypnotized can be hypnotized.

CAN I GET TRAPPED IN A HYPNOTIC TRANCE?

No! Everyone comes out of a trance. Hypnosis is a completely natural state, one that many of us experience in everyday life. For example, have you ever been driving in your car and all of a sudden realized that you missed your exit by several miles? Have you ever caught yourself daydreaming at work? Have you ever gotten so engrossed in a book that you didn't realize how much time you'd spent reading? These are all forms of hypnotic trances.

CAN I BE FORCED TO DO EMBARRASSING THINGS?

No! You are always in control of your behavior when you are in a hypnotic trance. You will not do things that you wouldn't normally do or that go against your core values while under hypnosis.

IS HYPNOSIS LIKE BEING ASLEEP?

Hypnosis promotes deep relaxation and an altered state of perception, but it does not put you to sleep. If you sleep through a hypnotic exercise, it is not helping you with anything more than taking a nap.

WILL I REMEMBER WHAT HAPPENED?

Most people do, although not everyone, such as in the case of Jo-Ellen above. Hypnosis promotes a heightened sense of awareness, and most people are completely aware of what is happening at all times. After you come out of the hypnotic trance, most people will likely remember the session in vivid detail.

What It Is Like to Be Hypnotized: A Firsthand Account

If you really want to know what the hypnosis experience is like, take a look at the following firsthand account from one of my researchers, an admitted "chocoholic," who agreed to let me hypnotize her to help her overcome her addiction to sugar. We recorded her hypnosis session as part of a ten-CD audio program to go with my book *Unchain Your Brain: 10 Steps to Breaking the Addictions That Steal Your Life.* During the session, I made suggestions to help her and listeners curb cravings and boost self-control.

When I do hypnosis specifically for weight loss, some of the common hypnotic suggestions I give to patients include "Feel full faster," "Eat more slowly," "Savor and enjoy each bite of your food," "Visualize yourself at your ideal weight and body," and "See the behaviors you need to do to get the body you want."

Considering that I get so many questions about what it is like to be hypnotized, I asked her to write about the experience on my blog. Here is what she had to say:

> I've never been hypnotized before (unless you count the time I was asked to come up onstage by Pat the Hip Hypnotist who used to perform on the Sunset Strip back in the seventies and eighties), so I was a little nervous when Dr. Amen told me he wanted to hypnotize me so listeners could follow along on the *Unchain Your Brain* audio program.
>
> A few ANTs started racing through my head: What if I say something embarrassing while in the hypnotic trance? What if I can't be hypnotized and I ruin the program? What if he makes me do something stupid?
>
> The ANTs melted away as soon as we got started with the process. I just listened to his soothing voice and let him take me on a beautiful journey.
>
> Soon the room we were in and the chair I was sitting in disappeared, and I was walking down a long staircase toward a beautiful park and a warm healing pool. I could still feel my body, and it felt warm, relaxed, and very light as if I was floating on air. I had expected to feel sleepy, but that wasn't the case at all. I actually felt very focused and alive, exploring this wondrous new world with all of my senses.
>
> I had always assumed that when you were under hypnosis, you

wouldn't know what the hypnotist was saying to you or remember any-thing about it afterward. But during the trance, I was very aware of every-thing Dr. Amen was saying and remembered everything about it later.

During the session Dr. Amen gave suggestions to help me kick my per-sonal addiction—sugar—while addressing other addictions for listeners.

After coming out of the trance, I felt a sense of calm relaxation. He asked me how long I thought the session had lasted and I told him about seven or eight minutes. He told me it was actually twenty-seven minutes! And I didn't move a muscle the entire time! For a fidgeter like me, that's amazing.

Overall, it was a wonderful experience! I certainly didn't need to feel nervous about it and my ANTs were all completely unfounded. But will it help me stay away from the cookies and candy? We'll see, but I did go home that night and toss out the M&M's that were in the kitchen cupboard.

You can find the *Unchain Your Brain* CD program as well as other hyp-nosis CDs and downloads that I have created for you on our website (www.amenclinics.com). You can use these CDs to help you go into a hypnotic trance anytime, anywhere (just *not* while you are driving)!

Practice Guided Imagery and Self-Hypnosis

Guided imagery and self-hypnosis are both great ways to boost your focus and self-control so you can stay on track with your weight-loss efforts. With guided imagery, like listening and following along to the hypnosis sessions on my CDs, someone else is inducing the hypnotic trance. With self-hypnosis, you are putting yourself in a hypnotic trance and can stay in the trance for as little or as long as you would like.

Learning self-hypnosis is easy. I have taught thousands of people how to do it successfully. It just takes a little practice. And the more you practice, the easier it will get. Now I'm going to show you how to do self-hypnosis to put yourself in a hypnotic trance. This exercise helps promote directed focus as well as stress relief, which are both critical to long-term weight-loss success.

SELF-HYPNOSIS EXERCISE

Use this self-hypnosis exercise on a regular basis.

- First, find a spot on the wall a little bit above your eye level and focus on it. (If you're lying down, find a spot on the ceiling so your eyes are looking up.) What this does is take all the outside distractions and helps you narrow your focus.

- Slowly count to twenty.

- Let your eyes close. As your eyes close, take three very deep, very slow breaths with your belly. As you do that, say to yourself with each inhalation, "I breathe in relaxation and warmth." With each exhale, say, "I blow out all the tension, all the worries, all the things that interfere with me becoming relaxed."

- After that third breath, keep breathing slowly and deeply, and with your eyes closed, roll them up as far as they'll go. What you're doing right now is tensing the tiny muscles of your eyes.

- After you roll them up as far as they'll go, let them come back down, and you'll notice that those muscles you tensed are now becoming relaxed. Just imagine the relaxation spreading from the top of your head all the way down to the bottom of your feet in a very slow progressive fashion.

- Now imagine yourself walking down a staircase or walking down a road, or going down an escalator. Something is moving you downward, making your body feel even more relaxed. As you walk down a staircase or descend on the escalator, count backward from ten.

- When you reach the number one, find yourself in your favorite place—a special place where you can go to anytime you need it in your imagination. For me, it would be the beach. For you, it might be the green forest or the snowy mountains. What is your special place that has relaxation written all over it? If you could go anyplace in the world, where would you go? Write the name of it here.

- Now I want you to go to that place and experience it in your mind with all five of your senses to see what's there, feel what's there, to hear what's there, and to smell and taste what's there. Stay in your special place for a few minutes.

- When you feel ready, walk back to the staircase or escalator and start heading back up slowly.

- When you reach the top of the staircase or escalator, open your eyes, and you should feel calm, refreshed, and alert.

Like to Dislike: Using the Power of Your Unconscious Mind to Eliminate Problem Foods

At Amen Clinics, I am blessed to work with some of the nation's best and most innovative psychiatrists. One of them is Larry Momaya, M.D., who is a master practitioner of a powerful technique called Like to Dislike, which is a technique in neurolinguistic programming (NLP). The basic concept is simple: you take a food that you know isn't good for you but can't stop eating and replace the way you encode that food in your brain with something you can't stand. Here are a few examples of how successful Like to Dislike can be.

Derek was an impulsive overeater who had attention deficit hyperactivity disorder and a real problem with chocolate. He had absolutely no control over his desire to eat chocolate. For example, he would be driving down the freeway, and all of a sudden he would get an urge for chocolate so intense that he would have to pull off the highway, stop at a gas station, buy a chocolate bar, and eat it right there on the side of the road.

Derek did one Like to Dislike session during which Dr. Momaya guided him to replace all the wonderful qualities he loved so much about chocolate with the thing he hated most—celery. At the end of the very first session, Dr. Momaya presented Derek with some gourmet chocolates and asked him if he had any desire to eat them.

Derek said, "No."

Dr. Momaya put the chocolates in Derek's hand and asked, "What do you feel like doing?"

"Nothing."

"Do you feel like eating this?"

"No."

"What do you want to do with it?"

"Throw it out."

How did Dr. Momaya know that Derek wasn't faking it? His body language spoke volumes about what he was really thinking. When he was handed the chocolates, Derek actually recoiled from them, a telling sign that he was repulsed by it.

Dr. Momaya also did a Like to Dislike session for one of the participants in our pilot weight-loss group. He led the session in front of about fifty people as a demonstration. This guy loved cheeseburgers. I mean really loved them. And he knew he needed to stop eating them in order to get his weight under control. Dr. Momaya guided him through the steps to make him associate cheeseburgers with the food he hated most—fish. His reaction was so strong that at the end of the session, he asked for a wastebasket because he thought he might get sick. Since that time, he hasn't eaten a single cheeseburger.

Dr. Momaya worked with one of our staff members on her love of bagels. At the end of the session, she said it had no effect on her. Three months later, however, she had not had any bagels. Other people have gone to Dr. Momaya to help them stop eating chips, candy, and frozen yogurt. He helped me with Rocky Road ice cream, which I have avoided since our work together. Dr. Momaya himself worked with another NLP practitioner to get rid of his own personal weakness: sweet potato fries. "When I went out to lunch, I just couldn't say no to the sweet potato fries," Dr. Momaya said. "I knew they weren't good for me, but I felt the need to order them instead of a side salad." The Like to Dislike process worked, and he hasn't eaten any sweet potato fries since October 2009.

GET SMART TO GET THINNER

"With my stress levels, I find that if I take the time to meditate every day in the morning, it is renewing for my mind and soul."

—Brandi

As part of my Like to Dislike session with Dr. Momaya, I thought about a bowl of Rocky Road ice cream and then changed the image of it to have the innate qualities (look and feel) of a food I can't stand—Brussels sprouts. It turned my desire away from Rocky Road ice cream for sure. If you are considering Like to Dislike with a therapist, look for a master practitioner of NLP like Dr. Momaya who has a lot of experience with this technique.

In addition, think carefully about the food you want to avoid and don't choose something that's too broad. For example, you wouldn't want to avoid "sugar" because sugar is in so many things, including brain healthy foods like fruit and low-fat yogurt—even unsweetened yogurt contains some natural sugars—and you may have a negative reaction to all of them. This helpful technique works best if you choose something very specific and if you have a very strong negative reaction to the food that you hate.

Meditate to Sharpen Your Focus and Stay on Track

Need a little assistance staying focused on your weight-loss plan? Meditation can help. Decades of research have shown that meditation (and prayer) benefits the brain in many ways that can make it easier for you to stick with your weight-loss program. Here's how.

MEDITATION ENHANCES FOCUS AND SUPERCHARGES ENERGY WHILE STRENGTHENING YOUR BRAIN'S BRAKE.

At the Amen Clinics, we performed a SPECT study on a Kundalini yoga form of meditation called Kirtan Kriya in which we scanned eleven people on one day when they didn't meditate and then the next day during a meditation session. The brain imaging scans taken after meditation indicated significant increases in activity in the prefrontal cortex (PFC), which shows that meditation helps people tune in, not out.

Researchers from other labs around the world have also demonstrated that meditation enhances activity in the brain's PFC, even to the point of boosting the numbers of brain cells. The better your PFC functions, the more focused and energetic you feel and the less impulsive you are. That helps you stick with your brain healthy eating program, pumps you up to exercise more, and increases your self-control so you can say no to the giant tub of buttered popcorn at the movies.

Strengthening the PFC can be tremendously beneficial for all brain types but is especially helpful for Type 2 Impulsive Overeaters and Type 3 Impulsive-Compulsive Overeaters.

MEDITATION IMPROVES EMOTIONAL STABILITY AND GIVES YOU A BIGGER BRAIN.

A 2009 brain imaging study performed at UCLA found that people who meditate on a regular basis have more gray matter in the hippocampus, orbito-frontal cortex, thalamus, and left inferior temporal gyrus than non-meditators. These areas are all involved in emotional regulation, which may explain why meditators tend to have more positive emotions and better control over their emotions. Keeping your emotions in check helps keep your eating in check, especially for Type 4 Sad or Emotional Overeaters.

MEDITATION REDUCES DEPRESSION.

Meditation improves your sense of psychological well-being and diminishes symptoms of depression. One study used EEG to show that people who meditated for eight weeks experienced changes in cerebral electrical activity that are typically associated with experiencing positive or joyful feelings.

MEDITATION REDUCES STRESS, SOOTHES ANXIETY,
AND FOSTERS RELAXATION.

Brain imaging studies have shown that meditation calms the anterior cingulate and basal ganglia, which diminishes worries and provides a sense of relaxation. A wealth of research indicates that people who meditate regularly have lower levels of stress, anxiety, and worry. Considering that stress is one of the most common triggers for overeating, reducing your stress levels can be vital to changing your eating patterns. The same is true for people who eat to calm anxiety, like our Type 5 Anxious Overeaters.

GET SMART TO GET THINNER

"I used to eat without thinking and didn't even realize I was eating. Now I'm more thoughtful of what I'm eating, and it tastes better. I'm eating less but enjoying it more."

—Carmen

MEDITATION MAKES YOU MORE MINDFUL.

Being mindful means paying attention to what you are doing, thinking, and feeling in the present moment. This is especially important for those of you who camp out on the couch all evening and devour entire bags of chips, pretzels, or cookies without even realizing it. With mindless eating, it's usually quantity over quality. You don't necessarily enjoy what you're eating; you just keep wanting more.

By contrast, when you eat mindfully, you meditate on each bite of food and become aware of the smells, tastes, colors, and textures of your food. You learn to savor each bite. This helps you become more aware of feeling full and stopping before you overeat. In a study on the effects of mindfulness on binge eating, a group of 18 women diagnosed with binge-eating disorder decreased their number of weekly binges from four to fewer than two. Fourteen of the women reduced their bingeing so much that they would no longer have met the criteria for binge-eating disorder.

My friend Andy Newberg, M.D., at the University of Pennsylvania, and his collaborator Mark Waldman, a therapist and associate fellow at the Center for Spirituality and the Mind at the University of Pennsylvania, have teamed up to do a SPECT brain study on mindful eating. At this writing, the study is in its earliest stages, and Andy is hesitant to report any specific findings. But he did say that the initial brain scans show that "the brain is different when eating mindfully." That doesn't surprise me at all.

MEDITATION MAKES YOU SMARTER.

Dharma Singh Khalsa, M.D., of the Alzheimer's Research and Prevention Foundation and Andy Newberg conducted a research study that was published in 2010 using brain SPECT imaging to evaluate the effects of meditation on memory in fifteen people with memory problems owing to normal aging or Alzheimer's disease. The group underwent a series of tests at the study's debut and again after meditating every day for eight weeks. The results showed that after the two months of daily meditation, the group's cerebral blood flow had increased in areas involved in retrieving memories. They also performed better on standardized tests that evaluate memory, cognition, and attention. Having a better memory is essential to help you remember all the important things you need to do in order to reach your weight-loss goals.

MEDITATION AIDS IN THE TREATMENT OF SUBSTANCE ABUSE.

If you are wondering what this has to do with helping you lose weight, remember that from my perspective, chronic overeating or bingeing is a form of substance abuse.

OVERVIEW OF THE MEDITATION BENEFITS FOR THE FIVE TYPES OF OVEREATERS

- **Type 1 Compulsive Overeaters** Meditation lowers activity in the anterior cingulate gyrus, which reduces compulsivity.
- **Type 2 Impulsive Overeaters** Meditation increases activity in the PFC, which improves focus, attention, and planning. It also boosts your self-control and lowers impulsivity.

- **Type 3 Impulsive-Compulsive Overeaters** See benefits for Types 1 and 2 above.

- **Type 4 Sad or Emotional Overeaters** Meditation decreases depression, which can reduce your desire to self-medicate your feelings of sadness or emptiness. It also boosts areas of the brain that regulate emotion, making you less vulnerable to emotional eating.

- **Type 5 Anxious Overeaters** Meditation cools overactive basal ganglia, which reduces your anxiety and lessens your need to eat as a way to comfort yourself.

Learning to Meditate Is Easy

You don't need to devote big chunks of time to the practice of meditation for stress relief or go to India for three months. In my clinical practice, I often recommend meditation as an integral part of a treatment plan. Many of my patients have reported back that they feel calmer and less stressed after just a few minutes of daily meditation.

GET SMART TO GET THINNER

"I do the saa-taa-naa-maa meditation before I get out of bed in the morning."
—Suzie

The following meditation exercises are effective, feel-good techniques to reset your nervous system so that you feel ever so much more relaxed. It is very powerful. You can do this whenever you feel stressed, anxious, or sad. For example, you can close your office door and take an inner journey on your lunch break. You can do this to mellow out after a hard day or after your children have gone to bed. I have even practiced guided imagery and self-hypnosis while sitting on trains, buses, and airplanes.

To help you get the most out of mediation, use the following tips and techniques.

PREPARE TO MEDITATE

- Find a quiet place that's free of distractions. Lock the door to avoid interruptions and turn off your cell phone.

- Give yourself twelve minutes to meditate, once or twice a day, preferably before breakfast and dinner, and don't stop until this time is up. Check a clock occasionally, or use a soft alarm, not a harsh one, as it might shock you out of your relaxation.

- Sit comfortably and consciously relax all your muscles from the bottom of your feet to the top of your head, and close your eyes. Enjoy your calm attitude as you breathe slowly and deeply from your belly.

- Try to forget all the thoughts that swirl through your mind. Put a stop to your internal monologue. Cease thinking in words. This is often the hardest part about meditation for people who are new to the practice. When memories arise, simply tell them to go away or imagine a broom gently sweeping them out of your mind. With practice, you will find that your thoughts become less intrusive.

DAILY TWELVE-MINUTE KIRTAN KRIYA MEDITATION PRACTICE

This twelve-minute meditation involves chanting the following simple sounds—"saa" "taa" "naa" "maa"—while doing repetitive finger movements. Do this every day for maximum effect.

- Touch the thumb of each hand to the index finger while chanting "saa."
- Touch the thumb of each hand to the middle finger while chanting "taa."
- Touch the thumb of each hand to the ring finger while chanting "naa."
- Touch the thumb of each hand to the pinkie finger while chanting "maa."
- Repeat the sounds for two minutes aloud.
- Repeat the sounds for two minutes whispering.
- Repeat the sounds for four minutes silently.
- Repeat the sounds for two minutes whispering.
- Repeat the sounds for two minutes aloud.
- When you finish, sit quietly for a minute or two, and try to merge your calmed mind and body with your regular mode of being.

I realize that many people are busy and some days, you just can't find the time to meditate for twelve minutes. Or when you are first trying meditation, you may find it difficult to focus your mind for twelve minutes. In either case, you may want to try something called the Relaxation Response developed

Kirtan Kriya Fingertip Movements

by Herbert Benson, M.D., at Harvard Medical School. This is a very simple introduction to meditation. I have found that many of my patients have managed to see benefits with just two minutes of meditation a day.

TWO-MINUTE RELAXATION RESPONSE MEDITATION

This two-minute meditation will help quiet your mind.

- Sit quietly.
- Close your eyes.
- Take slow deep breaths.
- Say the word *one* whenever you exhale.
- If your mind wanders, just bring your thoughts back to the word *one* as you exhale.

The Amen Solution All-Stars: Roy

At 6'7" Roy was an imposing force as an offensive tackle for the San Francisco 49ers. But in his second season, a knee injury put a swift end to his football career. Although his playing days were cut short, Roy had the privilege of seeing his son and then his grandson each carry on the family football tradition as professional players. All three of them joined our football player study as our only three-generation football family.

When Roy, now age seventy-three, first came to see us, he weighed 334 pounds. When I told Roy that I wanted him to weigh 225 pounds, he told

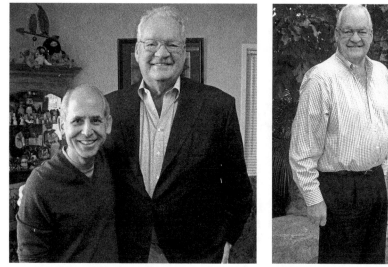

Before, 334 pounds   Six months later, 306 pounds

me, "My bones weight 225 pounds!" Then he started to negotiate with me. "How about 275?" he asked. We finally settled on a goal of 265.

Getting Roy motivated was easy. All he needed to hear was that the more overweight you are, the smaller your brain becomes. Roy runs a highly successful firm that conducts research and supports families in the transition of wealth from one generation to the next, so having a smaller brain was not an option for him. He was very motivated to have the best brain possible.

To boost his brain and trim his waistline, Roy began measuring his food and counting his calories and discovered that he had been eating far more than he realized. To cut down on calories, he traded his usual glass of wine with dinner for green tea. He finds that he gets just as much enjoyment out of the green tea, and he has much more energy in the evenings, which allows him to be more productive.

Once an inconsistent exerciser, he committed to a daily workout regimen that includes riding the recumbent bike, three hundred crunches, strength training, and stretching. He sets the alarm for 4:30 a.m. to get to the gym by 5 a.m., which he admits his wife isn't too happy about. Then he works out for an hour to an hour and a half and still gets to the office by about 8 a.m.

Meditation is also part of Roy's early morning routine. Roy has been meditating for about thirty years to help him focus and be present in the moment. "It's amazing how being present can create such a change in your whole body. The relaxation it creates in your body is magical," he said.

Roy's brain-boosting regimen also includes a daily handful of supplements that all of the players in our NFL study are taking. They include a high-quality multivitamin (our NeuroVite), fish oil (our Omega-3 Power), and our Brain & Memory Power Boost. He thinks these supplements are playing a major role in his sense of heightened brainpower, his weight-loss success, and his renewed vigor.

After about six months on our program, he has already lost 28 pounds and feels better than ever. "My wife complains that I have too much energy now. She says, 'You have the energy you had when you were forty.'"

Roy isn't the only one in the family who is reaping the benefits of better brain health. His son and grandson have each dropped about 40 pounds since beginning the program. And proving that a brain healthy lifestyle can be contagious, his wife is also losing weight by adopting some of Roy's new habits.

10

BUST YOUR BARRIERS

OVERCOME THE PEOPLE, PLACES, AND THINGS THAT SABOTAGE SUCCESS

Eileen, one of our All-Stars, was doing great with our weight-loss program and was thrilled to see the pounds melting away as she adopted brain healthy eating habits. But then she took a trip to Las Vegas and had to eat at one of those opulent buffets that Vegas is known for. You know the kind of buffet I'm talking about—fried foods galore, mashed potatoes smothered in butter, rich cream sauces on everything, and endless desserts. With these tempting foods right in front of her face, Eileen could have easily piled 5,000 calories—or more—onto her plate.

Riz, our Amen Clinics psychiatrist All-Star, had no problem sticking with his new eating regimen until he went to dinner parties with friends and family. Then his loved ones would offer him all kinds of foods that he used to love but that no longer fit into his new brain healthy lifestyle. Riz's friends and family would try to pressure him and coax him into eating or drinking things he had given up. "What's wrong with you?" they would ask. "You're not obese. Why aren't you having any kebab? Why aren't you eating any rice? You've always loved kebab and rice." They made Riz feel like he was being rude if he didn't give in and take a helping . . . or two.

Jeanne, sixty-five, is one of our weight-loss participants who lost 8 pounds in our ten-week program and then went on to lose another 32 for a total of 40 pounds in less than six months. She has learned to control her eating and curb her calories, but she says her husband occasionally tries to sabotage her. She says that even though he says he wants her to continue losing weight, he sometimes tries to get her to eat more than she should. "For breakfast, he'll give me two pieces of toast, two poached eggs, three pieces of turkey sausage, and a big glass of orange juice. I don't need all that, and I don't want it," she said.

I know that feeling very well. When I became a grandfather for the first time, I couldn't wait to visit my new grandson, Elias. When I went to my daughter's home, a friend of mine was also visiting. She asked me if I wanted something to eat, and I said no, I wasn't hungry. A few minutes later, she asked me again, and I told her no again. I thought that would be the end of that discussion, but she continued to ask me an additional five times if I wanted something to eat!

I call these people food pushers. And as you embark on your weight-loss journey, you need to be aware that on a daily basis, you will face many types of food pushers who will attempt to derail your weight-loss efforts. But food pushers are not the only obstacle you will face. Energy zappers that rob you of the will to exercise and money concerns that hold you back from getting healthy can also stand in the way of your efforts to improve your brain health and drop the extra weight. Sticking with your lifestyle changes isn't going to be smooth sailing, but if you are prepared for the challenges, you can deal with them more effectively.

Fortunately, Eileen, Riz, Jeanne, and I have all strengthened our brain's brake, which helps us say no when food pushers put us to the test. And we have learned to deal with the daily obstacles that threaten to derail us. Now it is your turn to learn how to fight back against the food pushers, energy zappers, and other obstacles. Do not let other people, places, or things make you fat, stupid, and unhappy!

Put a HALT to the Barriers to Weight Loss

The acronym HALT is a term commonly used in addiction treatment programs that can be very helpful in dealing with the daily obstacles you

---

GET SMART TO GET THINNER

"I used to always get sucked into buying popcorn at the movies. Now I bring my own snacks—a few cherries and walnuts with a bottle of water."

—Mario

will face. I understand that you may not equate an addiction program with weight loss, but as I have said before, chronic overeating is akin to substance abuse. And HALT has proven to be a very effective way to keep people on track when they are trying to change their habits. HALT stands for:

- Don't get too **hungry.** Eat frequent, small, high-quality meals and take nutritional supplements to optimize your brain, balance your blood sugar, and keep calories under control. See chapter 3 for more on brain healthy eating.

- Don't get too **angry.** Maintain control over your emotions and don't let negative thinking patterns keep you stuck in your old ways. See chapter 8 for more details on changing your thinking.

- Don't get too **lonely.** Social skills and a positive social network are critical to happiness and to freeing you from emotional overeating. Enlist a team of supporters and healthy role models.

- Don't get too **tired.** Make sleep a priority to boost brain function, moods, and energy levels, and to improve judgment and self-control.

Don't Let Food Pushers Sabotage Your Weight Loss

Food pushers are all around us. Every day, we're bombarded with the wrong messages about food. TV commercials, billboards, and radio ads are constantly showing us images of happy, attractive people enjoying greasy fast food, judgment-impairing cocktails, and dehydrating caffeinated drinks that decrease brain function and lower your self-control.

GET SMART TO GET THINNER

"The other night, my friends brought out some ice cream and cookie thing. I told myself they're not going to stop you, you're going to have to stop yourself so just turn the other way. And I did."

—Eva

Corporate America is highly skilled at pushing people to eat and drink things that are not good for brain health. Restaurants and fast-food joints train employees to "upsell" as a way to increase sales and, subsequently, expand our waistlines. Here are some of the sneaky tactics food sellers use to try to get you to eat and drink more.

- Do you want to supersize that for only thirty-nine cents?
- Do you want fries with your meal?
- Do you want bread first? (This makes you hungrier so you eat more!)
- Do you want an appetizer?
- Do you want another drink?
- Do you want a larger drink? It is a better deal!

Your response to all of these questions should be no! Eating or drinking more than you need, just because it's cheaper, will cost you far more in health care problems in the long run.

GET SMART TO GET THINNER

"I have friends who actually told me I was being rude because I said no thank you to the food they were offering me. It was hard at first, but now they know not to offer it to me."

—Derek

Your beloved friends and family can also make you fat—if *you* let them. A 2007 study published in the *New England Journal of Medicine* found that your chances of becoming obese increase dramatically if you have friends and family who become obese, regardless of how far away they live. Even if friends live hundreds of miles apart, they can still have a strong impact on your weight. For this study, the researchers repeatedly evaluated the BMI of 12,067 people over a thirty-two-year period. They found that having an obese pal increased the risk for obesity by 57 percent and added an average of seventeen pounds to one's frame. Having an obese sibling raised the risk by 40 percent, and having an obese spouse increased it by 37 percent.

Friends also play a major role in influencing the eating habits of tweens and teens. A 2009 study in the *American Journal of Clinical Nutrition* tested the snacking habits of twenty-three overweight and forty-two healthy weight young people. Results showed that the young folks gobbled up substantially more snacks when they were with a friend compared with when they were with a peer they didn't know. Also, when an overweight kid ate with a friend who was also plump, he consumed about 300 calories more than if he ate with a healthy weight friend.

So, is obesity contagious? To a certain extent, I would have to say yes. As I like to say, you are who you eat with. If you surround yourself with people who have bad brain habits, it is easy to get sucked into those habits. In most cases, your friends and family inadvertently influence you to adopt their bad habits. Sometimes, however, they may willfully try to undermine your efforts.

GET SMART TO GET THINNER

"Lose weight slowly and consistently to build new habits and a new way of life."

—Jamie

When you start living a brain healthy life and losing weight, it can make those around you uncomfortable, especially if they are overweight or have a lot of bad brain habits of their own. Deep down, some people—even those who love you the most—don't want you to succeed because it will make them feel like more of a failure.

For others, their habits are so ingrained that they simply don't know how to react to your new lifestyle. Many of my patients notice this kind of behavior with their families, friends, and coworkers. For example, a friend who smokes may thoughtlessly light up in front of you even though you are trying to quit. A neighbor might show up with a box of home-cooked brownies for your birthday when you are trying to curb your sugar intake. At work, the receptionist may bring in doughnuts and coffee for your company meetings, or your supervisor may invite your team to go to happy hour for some high-calorie cocktails.

GET SMART TO GET THINNER

"When I started eating brain healthy foods, my wife really got into it too. She's losing weight also and is below her magic point for the first time in twenty-five years."

—Bob

On the flip side, your new brain healthy habits may rub off on your friends and family. When people see the new and improved you, they may be inspired to get on the brain healthy bandwagon. Take Riz, for example.

His friends who were somewhat offended when he first started turning down food are now asking him for tips on how to lose weight.

The people around you can either hurt or help your chances for success. This is why it is so important to encourage the people in your social network to get on board with your brain healthy weight-loss efforts.

When you enlist your friends, family, and coworkers to support you in your new brain healthy lifestyle, they will be less likely to put you in situations that jeopardize your weight loss. It is also critical to create a strong support group of like-minded brain healthy role models, such as our online community, where you can turn for help when you need it.

People aren't the only pushers. Places and environmental cues can trigger your cravings and overeating. Almost everywhere you go, you will see reminders of the foods you used to crave or that you ate mindlessly. Drive to work, and you'll have to pass by the fast-food place where you used to order three cheeseburgers, jumbo fries, and an all-you-can-drink soda. Take a cruise to Alaska because you want to see the beautiful scenery, and you'll have to face unbelievably copious amounts of food and desserts at the buffet, not to mention the free-flowing alcohol.

Even though churches can be very good for your soul, many of them can be terrible for your waistline. I have gone to church my whole life and lately have been frustrated by the generally poor food they serve their parishioners. Recently, I went to church near my home. My wife, Tana, dropped our daughter off at children's church and I went to get us our seats. As I walked in I passed the doughnuts for sale for a dollar apiece, men were cooking sausage and bacon, and I saw hundreds of hot dog buns stacked up for after the service. I was so irritated that when my wife joined me she saw me making notes to myself on my BlackBerry. Giving me one of those disapproving looks that only she can give me about typing on my BlackBerry in church, I showed her what I had typed in: "Go to church and get dollar doughnuts, sausage, bacon, hot dogs . . . Send people to heaven early. They need to know how to become a brain healthy church." Tana agreed and forgave my indiscretion. Work to help your church, school, business, and family become a brain healthy place.

GET SMART TO GET THINNER

"Most people want to lose weight fast, but then it fails. The whole point is if you just tweak a few things, you can lose a pound a week and be successful."

—Diane

See chapter 6 for more information on how to deal with the urges that arise from environmental cues.

FOOD PUSHERS YOU MAY HAVE TO FACE

TV commercials	County fairs
Billboards	Amusement parks
Radio ads	Brownies selling cookies
Servers in restaurants	Little Leaguers selling
Cashiers in fast-food outlets	candy bars
Spouses	Vendors offering free samples
Parents	Friends
Grandparents	Neighbors
In-laws	Bosses
Kids	Coworkers
Churches	Vending machines at
AA organizations	work/school
Community clubs	Office/school cafeteria
Gyms	Teachers
Holidays	Classmates
Movie theaters	Students
Sports arenas	School administrators

Learning to deal with and say no to all of these pushers in the home, on the town, at work, and at school is critical to your success. Here are some tips to help you fight back.

FIFTY TIPS FOR DEALING WITH FOOD PUSHERS

1. Ask your spouse and kids to hide unhealthy treats and snacks out of view or get rid of them so you don't have to be tempted.
2. If you are going to a dinner with friends or family, call ahead to inform the host that you are on a special brain healthy diet and won't be able to eat certain foods. You only have to do this once or twice before your friends start to ask you what they could serve that is brain healthy.
3. If you are at a business luncheon, and your new boss or a potential client raves about how wonderful the bread is and offers it to you, take one small bite, tell them it is delicious, and then wait for your meal.

4. When going to parties, consider eating something at home first so you won't be hungry at the event.

5. Be up front with food pushers. Explain that you are trying to eat a more balanced diet and that when they offer you cake, chips, or pizza, it makes it more difficult for you.

6. Instead of going out to lunch or dinner with friends, choose activities that aren't centered around food, such as going for a walk.

7. If your coworkers invite you to happy hour, but you don't want them to push you to drink alcohol, ask the bartender to put sparkling water in a glass with a splash of cranberry juice and sip it slowly.

8. When people offer seconds, tell them you are pleasantly full. If they insist, explain that you are trying to watch your calories. If they continue to push extra helpings on you, gently ask them why they are bent on sabotaging your efforts to be healthy.

9. I know some people who will accept a piece of cake or a cocktail and then toss it in the trash or the sink as soon as the host turns away.

10. Avoid visiting with coworkers who have a bowl of candy on their desk.

11. Tell your host you don't drink alcohol. Period.

12. With hosts you don't know well and likely won't see again, consider telling them you have food allergies so you don't have to try their chocolate mousse pie or mayonnaise-laden dip.

13. Eat very slowly so when the host starts asking guests if they want seconds, you can say you are still working on your first helping. By the time you have finished, the second round of eating could be over, and you won't have to be subjected to the offer for more.

14. Give kids a healthy sack lunch so they don't have to eat from the cafeteria, if schools serve unhealthy food.

15. Commit to taking control of your own body and don't let other people make you fat and stupid.

16. When food commercials come on TV, leave the room, switch stations, or hit the mute button.

17. When driving past food billboards, focus on how many calories are in the food they are offering and allow yourself to feel disgusted, because you know if you give in to it, you will be sitting in extra fat.

18. When food-related radio ads are aired, turn off the radio or switch to another station.
19. Tell restaurant servers "no bread" or "no chips" before you're seated.
20. Tell restaurant servers "no dessert" before they have a chance to bring the dessert tray to your table.
21. When ordering fast food, just say no to supersizing.
22. Ask your spouse not to eat trigger foods in front of you.
23. If family members are eating foods that tempt you, leave the room until they finish.
24. Inform parents and in-laws ahead of time that you won't be partaking in certain foods at family gatherings.
25. Ask grandparents to avoid giving food rewards to your children.
26. Don't buy junk food for your kids or keep it in the house for them. If they have it, you'll want it. And it's better for their brain health too.
27. Ask friends or your spouse to split an entrée with you.
28. Ask the restaurant server to pack up half your meal to go before they bring it to you.
29. If the neighbor brings you a plate of chocolate chip cookies, immediately "regift" them to someone else.
30. If the boss brings birthday cake for your birthday, say thank you, take one small bite, and tell them how wonderful it is.
31. If you can't resist those high-calorie cocktails or you're worried that a few glasses of wine will ruin your self-control for the rest of the evening, say no to happy hour with your coworkers.
32. Don't walk past the vending machines at work/school.
33. Take a sack lunch to work instead of eating out with coworkers.
34. When a coworker suggests celebrating birthdays with cupcakes, recommend a healthy alternative.
35. If coworkers want to share their snacks, say no thank you.
36. Ask office administrators to contract with healthy food providers and get rid of vending machines filled with sodas and candy.
37. At church, skip the doughnuts and coffee after the service and stand outside if you want to socialize.
38. At community clubs, bring your own snacks.
39. Don't take the free samples of the "energy bars" or "energy drinks" offered at the gym. Remember "energy" equals "calories."

40. At all-you-can-eat buffets, go for the salad (dressing on the side), steamed vegetables, and lean protein first; then, after you have eaten that, go back if you are still hungry and want to try a higher-calorie item. Chances are you will eat a much smaller portion than if you had started with the fatty fare.

41. Bring your own healthy snacks to the movies so you don't have to go near the concession stand.

42. If you're at a sporting event, be aware that many ballparks and sports arenas are offering healthier options, so explore all the offerings rather than heading straight for the hot dog vendor.

43. If you can't resist the goodies at county fairs or amusement parks, get one item and split it among your friends.

44. When temptation wins out, use the three-bite rule. Take three bites of the item, and then toss it.

45. Donate money to the Girl Scouts rather than buying cookies.

46. When your spouse asks you to finish off the small amount of food left over from dinner, say no, box it up, and put it in the fridge for another meal.

47. When it's your turn to host a party, send all the leftovers home with your guests so you won't be tempted to eat them.

48. If someone in your dining party orders fries for the table, make sure you have a glass of water or green tea to sip on while they munch. It will keep you occupied and help prevent you from reaching for a fry, or two, or twenty.

49. At the grocery store checkout stand, keep your eyes focused on the checker so you don't have to look at the candy and other impulse-buy items calling out to you.

50. Make it a rule *never* to take free food samples *anywhere*!

GET SMART TO GET THINNER

"I used to be around people who told me I was fat. I have taken charge of that and don't have critical people around me anymore. Now I've surrounded myself with people who express appreciation and encouragement. I didn't realize how others' negativity was affecting me."

—Laura

Hold the Bread Before Meals

Why do restaurants serve baskets of bread before each meal for free? Why not cheese? Why not almonds or chunks of beef or chicken? The reason is that bread makes you hungrier and encourages you to eat more. Bread, especially white bread made from bleached and processed flour, spikes your blood sugar and boosts the natural feel-good neurotransmitter serotonin in the brain. Serotonin helps you feel happier and less anxious.

On brain SPECT scans, I have seen that serotonin interventions help to relax or lower function in the prefrontal cortex (PFC). When I prescribe antidepressant medications or supplements that boost serotonin in the brain, my patients often say they feel better, but that they are also less motivated. Anything that lowers PFC function makes you more impulsive and less worried about long-term consequences. The bread or simple carbohydrate to start a meal helps you feel better but also more impulsive when the dessert tray comes by later on. Hold the bread, wait for your meal, and you will be happier with the end result.

The Three Circles: Know When You're Safe, When You're Vulnerable, and When You're in Danger

It is absolutely critical that you know what helps keep you on track with your weight loss, what makes you more likely to fall back into your old ways, and what puts you in imminent danger of overeating. To help my patients understand the people, places, and things that are helping them reach their goals and those that are putting them at greater risk for overeating, I use an exercise called the Three Circles.

For this exercise, I have my patients take a page, draw three circles on it, and label them "Red Circle," "Yellow Circle," and "Green Circle." In the green circle, I have them write down all the things that help them stay on track with their weight-loss and brain health goals. In the yellow circle, they put things that make them more vulnerable to getting off track. In the red circle, they list their danger zones—the things that put them in imminent danger of reverting back to their bad habits.

Following is an example of what the Three Circles might look like for someone who is a binge eater. Then there is a blank form called My Three Circles that you can use to identify what helps keep you safe, what makes you more vulnerable, and what puts you in danger. Keep this page with you to help remind you what's helping you reach your goals and what is putting you at risk. You can also find an interactive version of this exercise on our website.

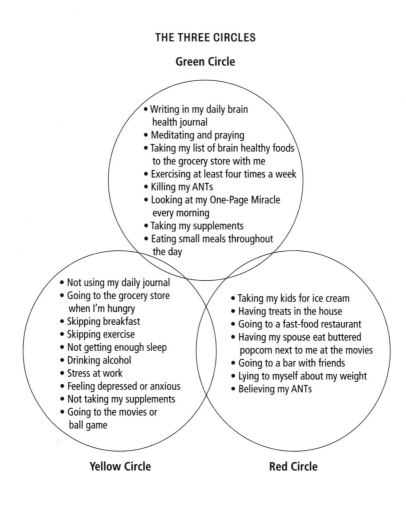

THE THREE CIRCLES

Green Circle

- Writing in my daily brain health journal
- Meditating and praying
- Taking my list of brain healthy foods to the grocery store with me
- Exercising at least four times a week
- Killing my ANTs
- Looking at my One-Page Miracle every morning
- Taking my supplements
- Eating small meals throughout the day

- Not using my daily journal
- Going to the grocery store when I'm hungry
- Skipping breakfast
- Skipping exercise
- Not getting enough sleep
- Drinking alcohol
- Stress at work
- Feeling depressed or anxious
- Not taking my supplements
- Going to the movies or ball game

- Taking my kids for ice cream
- Having treats in the house
- Going to a fast-food restaurant
- Having my spouse eat buttered popcorn next to me at the movies
- Going to a bar with friends
- Lying to myself about my weight
- Believing my ANTs

Yellow Circle   **Red Circle**

GET SMART TO GET THINNER

"When I eat things that aren't healthy, it makes me feel lethargic, and I don't want to go to the gym. In the past, I would have skipped it, but now I know that once I go to the gym, I will feel better. So even if I'm not feeling up to it, I go anyway."

—Monica

MY THREE CIRCLES

Green Circle

In this circle, write what helps keep you safe and on track with your weight-loss goals.

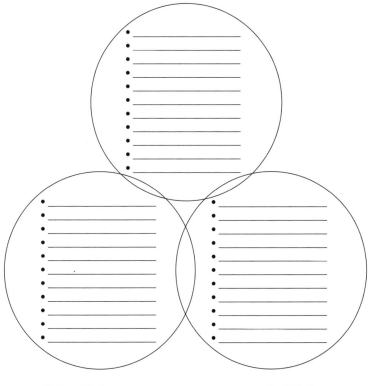

Yellow Circle

In this circle, write what makes you more vulnerable to reverting back to old habits.

Red Circle

In this circle, write what puts you in immediate danger of overeating or bingeing.

Don't Let Energy Zappers Prevent You from Getting the Exercise You Need

Maria, forty-four, is one of my patients who has started doing a thirty-minute burst routine every morning before work in an effort to burn calories and boost her brain. But several days a week, her husband, Ben, tries to coax her into staying in bed with him and going back to sleep instead of exercising.

Be prepared to deal with people who try to get in the way of your commitment to exercise. Like Maria, your spouse might tempt you to give up your workout in favor of a little extra shut-eye. You might be heading out the door to go to the gym when your kids say they need a ride somewhere *now.* Your boss might put a last-minute project on your desk just as you were about to leave work to go play basketball. Don't give in to these people. Slip out of bed quietly so your spouse can go back to sleep. Tell your kids you will give them a ride after you have worked out. And let your boss know you had a prior commitment, but you will work on the new project later that night.

When an energy zapper tries to keep you from exercising, let them know why exercise is important to you and why it is also beneficial to them. Arm yourself with responses like these:

> *"I'm exercising because it makes me feel good and helps keep me healthy by preventing cravings. If you care about me and my health, you won't ask me to skip it."*
> *"Physical activity puts me in a better mood, which will help our relationship and make me a better partner/friend."*
> *"If I go exercise for an hour, I will think much more clearly afterward and will do a better job on this project."*

The people around you aren't the only energy zappers. There are many other things that will rob you of energy, including:

- Inherited brain disorders
- Infectious causes
- Hormonal issues
- Anemia
- Brain trauma
- Environmental toxins
- Many medications
- Chronic stress
- Untreated past emotional trauma
- Caffeine
- Smoking
- Poor eating habits
- Poor sleep
- Too much alcohol
- Lack of exercise
- Low/erratic blood sugar states from any cause

Here are ways to boost your energy.

- Treat the energy robbers described above.
- Get at least seven hours of sleep.
- Eat a brain healthy diet.
- Maintain a level blood sugar.
- Exercise four to five times a week.
- Use stress-reduction techniques.
- Test and optimize hormone levels.
- Meditate.
- Eat low-calorie, high-fiber foods (fruits, vegetables, beans, and whole grains).
- Drink green tea, which includes theanine.
- Take natural supplements, such as ashwagandha and green tea leaf extract.

Sometimes your biggest energy zapper can be yourself—and your excuses. So many of us can come up with a million excuses why we shouldn't exercise. Even I have days when I have to engage in a full-fledged battle against my excuses to get out the door.

COMMON EXERCISE EXCUSES

- I'm too tired.
- I'm too busy.
- I'm too fat to go to a gym.
- I'm too old to exercise.
- I'm too stressed out.
- It's dark out.
- It's drizzling.
- It's too cold.
- I don't know what kind of exercises to do.
- I'm bored with my workout.
- I hate exercising.
- I'm already five minutes late for my aerobics class, so I may as well not go at all.
- I'm still sore from yesterday's workout.
- I'm not in the mood.

- I get enough exercise around the house.
- I don't have any exercise equipment.
- The gym is too far away.
- I can't leave the kids alone.

By now, you may recognize that these thoughts are ANTs that can drain your energy and motivation to exercise. If you find these thoughts creeping into your head, go back to chapter 8, and do the exercises to challenge them.

Don't Let Money Concerns Stand in the Way of Brain Health

Brooke, twenty-two, wants to optimize her brain so she can stop her sad and emotional overeating, and she knows that exercising and taking a multivitamin, fish oil, and vitamin D could help. But she's worried about the cost of a gym membership and high-quality supplements, so she doesn't get the mood-boosting exercise or nutrients she needs and continues to overeat.

GET SMART TO GET THINNER

"A lot of people think, 'I can't afford to eat fish,' but if you're only eating four ounces at twenty dollars a pound, you're only going to pay five dollars. You might be able to afford that."

—Nathan

Being too fat is what is really expensive. It can ruin your health and lead to serious diseases that can drain your brain and your bank account. Plus, research shows that being obese is associated with lower salaries and fewer job opportunities.

Fortunately, I can tell you that living a brain healthy life doesn't have to cost a bundle. In fact, many of the tips in this book are absolutely free. Just check the following list for inexpensive ways to boost your brain.

FIFTY FREE AND LOW-COST WAYS TO IMPROVE BRAIN HEALTH

1. Loving your brain is free.
2. Talking about the brain with family, friends, coworkers, and classmates is free.

3. Learning something from articles and TV features about the brain is free.

4. Keeping a daily journal to track your brain healthy habits is free.

5. Becoming aware of the various brain systems is free.

6. Understanding your own brain and how it affects your life is free.

7. Avoiding activities at high risk for brain injury is free.

8. Putting a halt to any drug use saves money.

9. Limiting your exposure to toxins like nail polish and hair chemicals is free.

10. Cooking healthy food at home can be less expensive than eating out.

11. Buying frozen fruits in bulk is an inexpensive way to get your antioxidants.

12. Buying frozen vegetables in bulk is another low-cost option.

13. Stocking up on brain healthy beans is an inexpensive way to get more fiber in your diet.

14. Skipping the candy, cookies, and ice cream lowers your food bill.

15. Eating fewer calories costs less.

16. Eating five or six small meals doesn't cost any more than eating three big meals.

17. Saying no to supersizing your meal saves money.

18. At restaurants, splitting meals cuts the check in half.

19. Skipping the appetizers and desserts lowers your check total.

20. Cutting out the alcohol can significantly reduce your dinner tab or bar tab.

21. Quitting smoking saves money spent on cigarettes.

22. Getting more sleep is free.

23. Drinking water costs less than drinking energy drinks, coffee, or sodas.

24. Exercising outdoors is free.

25. Thinking positive thoughts is free.

26. Cutting TV time is free.

27. Limiting video game playing is free.

28. Buying fewer video games saves money.

29. Reducing Internet time is free.

30. Limiting texting can save money.

31. Cutting caffeine can trim your Starbucks bill.

32. Getting books from the library for new learning is free.
33. Getting foreign language CDs from the library is free.
34. Games and puzzles are a low-cost investment for mental workouts.
35. Classes at local community colleges and the Learning Annex are relatively inexpensive.
36. Improving at your favorite activities can be free.
37. Shaking up your daily routine is free.
38. Surrounding yourself with smart people is free.
39. Meditation is free.
40. Prayer, which offers many of the same benefits as meditation, is free.
41. Saying no to invitations that don't serve your goals is free.
42. Being grateful is free.
43. Deep breathing for stress reduction is free.
44. Self-hypnosis is free.
45. Soothing music doesn't require a big investment.
46. Focusing on positive memories is free.
47. Talking back to your ANTs is free.
48. Writing down your goals is free.
49. Staying focused on what motivates you is free.
50. Saying no to food pushers who want you to eat unhealthy things is free.

On the other hand, there are times when it is well worth it to spend money on your brain health. Don't skimp when it comes to the following:

- Get a complete physical to check for medical conditions that might be affecting your weight and brain health.
- Take high-quality supplements to optimize your brain and control cravings.
- See a professional to diagnose and treat possible brain disorders.
- Choose a treatment program if you suffer from an eating disorder, such as bulimia.

When Your Brain Fights Change, Fight Back

Change is an uncomfortable process, and your brain is hardwired to resist change. When your brain tells you to stick with the same old habits that have made you fat, you need to fight back. The steps in this book are designed to help you rewire your brain so you can lose weight, but don't expect it to be as easy as flipping a switch. It takes time to overwrite old neural pathways with new ones. Here are a few tips that can help you retrain your brain to stay on the right path.

GET SMART TO GET THINNER

"It's the little changes that will help you get to your goal. A little tweak can make a big difference."

—Katrina

DON'T TRY TO CHANGE EVERYTHING AT ONCE.

If you have come to the decision that you want to make changes in your life, you probably want them to happen *now!* But after nearly thirty years of helping patients navigate the change process, I have learned that taking a gradual approach is the surest way to success. So many people try to change all at once, but this almost inevitably invites disappointment and failure. You don't have to change dozens of behaviors at once. Start with a few vital behaviors—the ones that will have the biggest immediate impact—and go from there.

BELIEVE YOU CAN DO IT.

If you don't believe in yourself, you will never achieve your goals. Take what you learned from chapter 8 and start changing your negative thinking patterns to honest and positive thinking to help you believe that you can do it.

REWARD YOURSELF FOR THE SMALL SUCCESSES.

When you reach short-term goals, give yourself a pat on the back, but don't celebrate with substances or activities that harm your brain. Why do we choose to celebrate birthdays, promotions, and other successes with foods and drinks that decrease brain function and make us fat? Find brain healthy ways that don't involve eating and drinking to reward yourself. Here are some non-food rewards you might want to try.

"I'm doing the program in steps. At first, I just tried to work on my eating and filling out the *Daily Journal*. Now I'm working on relaxation techniques."

—Kim

- Enjoy a few hours of quiet time.
- Spend an evening alone with a good book.
- Take a warm bath.
- Ask your significant other to give you a massage.
- Give yourself a manicure or pedicure or go to a nail salon.
- Make a hair appointment.
- Get a spa treatment.
- Go to the movies or watch a favorite movie on TV.
- Download your favorite songs to your iPod.
- Relax with your favorite magazine.
- Give yourself a compliment. Write it down and put it where you can see it often.
- Visit a museum.
- Listen to your favorite relaxation CD.
- Go dancing with your friends or significant other.
- Go hiking with a friend.
- Spend an afternoon playing fetch with your dog.
- Get some fresh-cut flowers, a plant, or herbs for the garden.
- Call a friend to share your success.
- Buy a spice rack for all the new spices you're using on your food.
- Get a new vegetable steamer or other kitchen gadget to make healthy cooking easier.
- Act like a kid—go fly a kite or play Frisbee with a friend.
- Treat yourself to a personal training session.
- Ask your spouse to take care of the kids for an entire day so you can do whatever you like.
- Buy some new workout clothes.
- Get a pedometer.
- Get a sports watch that also tracks your heart rate and calories burned.
- Spend time with a friend you haven't seen in a long time.
- Go out for a guys' night out.

GET SMART TO GET THINNER

"Every eight to ten days, I reward myself with something I love."

—Jeff

- Go out for a girls' night out.
- Go to a garage sale.
- Go window shopping.
- Go antiquing.
- Put on that bathing suit you refused to wear for so long and go swimming at the local pool.
- Take a day off work.
- Invite friends over for a game night.
- Go to a club where you can sing karaoke.
- Ask a friend to take photos of the new you.
- Donate your "fat" clothes to a local shelter.
- Hire someone to do the housework or gardening for a day so you can have more "me" time.
- Spend an afternoon at the beach showing off your new figure.
- Let yourself sleep in late on Sunday.
- Try a new fitness class.
- Go to a local sporting event, like a high school football game or baseball game.
- Take a day trip.
- Wear that sleeveless shirt you have never worn because your arms used to jiggle too much.
- Buy something for your favorite hobby—yarn for knitting, scrapbooking materials, or tools, for example.
- Buy yourself a number of small, inexpensive gifts and wrap them up in identical packages. When you reach one of your goals, unwrap one of them for a nice surprise.
- Put one dollar—or fifty cents or a dime—in a piggy bank each time you do a particular brain healthy habit. Let it add up until you reach a big goal and spend it on whatever you'd like.
- Give yourself a "Congratulations" certificate (you can create one on your computer) for every 5 or 10 pounds of weight loss. Keep them somewhere you can look at them often.

When should you reward yourself? It's up to you. Of course, you can reward yourself for every pound—or every 5 pounds—but rewarding yourself for the brain healthy habits that are going to help you shed those pounds may be a smarter move. After all, it's the new habits you want to reinforce.

For example, you can reward yourself for meditating every single day for a week. You can give yourself something special for doing your ANT exercises ten times. You can celebrate a week without caffeine, a month of eating vegetables every day, or exercising four times a week. In general, it's best to reward yourself for the habits that are the hardest to change.

DON'T SWAP ONE BAD HABIT FOR ANOTHER.

If you've got a sweet tooth, you may think that kicking your sugar habit is the ultimate goal. So instead of chomping on chocolate in the afternoon, you start sipping a diet soda or a café latte. No, it isn't chocolate, but it still isn't good for your brain or your weight-loss efforts. I see this so many times with my patients who quit one bad habit only to acquire another one in its place.

GET SMART TO GET THINNER

"I control my food now. My food doesn't control me."

—Lynda

Some people even turn to illicit drugs. At the 2010 meeting of the American Society of Metabolic and Bariatric Surgery, researchers presented evidence that some people who have bariatric surgery replace their food addiction with drug or alcohol addiction. A survey of post–bariatric surgery patients in substance abuse programs revealed that 85 percent of them put some of the blame on "addiction substitution" and 75 percent thought "unresolved psychological issues" played a role in their substance abuse.

This doesn't surprise me because, as I said in the introduction, stapling your stomach may be working on the wrong organ. There may be underlying biological, psychological, social, or spiritual causes for your overeating. If you get rid of your problem foods or have surgery to shrink your stomach but do *not* address these underlying problems, you won't make any progress.

You will simply look for other ways to self-medicate. To be your best self, you need to kick your bad habits without replacing them with others.

GET BACK ON TRACK—SETBACKS DON'T MEAN FAILURE.

The road to change is not a one-way street. The steps to change are not static. I frequently tell my patients that their journey will be like going up and down a staircase. They will go up several steps, feel like they've made progress, then go back down a few steps when difficult situations arise. They will make several more steps of progress, then slip back a few, but usually not as many as before. Usually, the slope of progress is in an upward, positive direction.

If you aren't expecting to encounter setbacks, it can derail your efforts. Let's say you've been doing a great job sticking to your daily calorie limit and have lost five pounds after a few weeks. But then you go to your parents' house for the holidays where you overindulge and end up gaining two pounds in a week. Then you feel like you've blown it, so you continue overeating after you return home and then you give up entirely on changing.

Understanding that setbacks are part of the process and planning how to deal with them makes them easier to handle. So you ate more than you should during the holidays and gained a couple pounds—just get back on your program the next day. Remember, losing weight is not a race, and faster is not necessarily better. Slow and steady is the healthiest way to lose weight and keep it off.

GET SMART TO GET THINNER

"You can't beat yourself up for the slipups. If you ate too much one day, just go for a longer walk the next day."

—Jesse

IF YOU HIT A PLATEAU, CHANGE THINGS UP A BIT.

Hitting a plateau can be one of the most frustrating challenges in your weight-loss journey. A plateau is when your scale seems to get stuck on a certain number and just won't budge even though you haven't veered away from your new brain healthy habits. Rest assured that this is a common scenario.

Often, the problem lies with your resting basal metabolic rate (BMR).

This is the number of calories you need to maintain your current weight. You see, when you lose weight, your BMR goes down too, so you need fewer calories to maintain your weight.

For example, let's say you are a fifty-year-old man who is 5'10" and 250 pounds, and you eat 3,000 calories a day. If you cut the recommended 500 calories per day from your diet to lose one pound a week, you'll be eating about 2,500 calories a day, and you'll start to see the weight come off. (To keep it simple for this example, we won't factor exercise into the mix.) If you lose 40 pounds in six months like some of our All-Stars, your BMR goes down and your body no longer burns as many calories per day. So the 2,500 calories you are still eating may actually be too high for you now.

Using the equation below, at 210 pounds and sedentary, you would need a total of 2,308 calories per day to maintain your weight. But you are still eating 2,500 calories, so the scale stops moving in the right direction. As you lose weight, you need to make adjustments to your caloric intake and energy output to compensate for your changing BMR.

BASAL METABOLIC RATE (BMR) EQUATION

Women: 655 + (4.35 x weight in pounds) + (4.7 x height in inches)—(4.7 x age in years)

Men: 66 + (6.23 x weight in pounds) + (12.7 x height in inches)—(6.8 x age in years)

Take that number and multiply by it by the appropriate number below:

1.2—if you are sedentary (little or no exercise)

1.375—if you are lightly active (light exercise/sports 1–3 days/week)

1.55—if you are moderately active (moderate exercise/sports 3–5 days/week)

1.75—if you are very active (hard exercise/sports 6–7 days a week)

1.9—if you are extra active (very hard exercise/sports and a physical job or strength training twice a day)

Total: _____

GET SMART TO GET THINNER

"I wanted to lose 2 to 3 pounds a week, but some weeks I only lost 1 pound. Don't get down on yourself when this happens. Be gentle with yourself. Praise yourself for what you have done rather than feeling bad because you think you haven't done enough."

—Al

The first thing you need to do when your scale gets stuck is make sure that you really have hit a plateau. Even if the number on the scale hasn't dropped, your body composition might still be improving. That is exactly what happened to Eileen, one of our All-Stars. After losing about 15 pounds in her first ten-week session and another 15 in her second ten-week session, her weight loss seemed to stall at about 4 pounds midway through her third session. But her body was still changing. In fact, even though she had only dropped 4 pounds, she had dropped two full pants sizes during her third session alone! Altogether she went down five pants sizes in about six months.

So don't automatically get discouraged if the number on the scale isn't changing fast enough for you. We often get so hung up on a specific number that we lose sight of our real goal, which is to look slimmer, feel happier and more energetic, and be smarter.

If you really have hit a plateau, then it is probably time to decrease your caloric intake and change up your workout routine. For example, let's say you have been doing thirty minutes of walking with bursts four times a week. At first, it was probably a real challenge for you. But after a while, your body learns to work more efficiently, and you no longer burn as many calories doing the same activity. Plus, as your body becomes lighter, you burn fewer calories.

To increase your calorie burn, you have to pump up the intensity of your workouts. Consider adding some hills, jogging, or full-out sprints to your walking routine. Or add fifteen minutes to your workouts. Or try doing another activity altogether, like swimming or dancing, which will challenge your muscles in new ways.

GET SMART TO GET THINNER

"I stopped believing that I couldn't do it."

—Sarah

It is also a good idea to add strength training to your routine because working your muscles ultimately boosts your metabolism. The more lean muscle mass you have, the higher your metabolism. Strength training can help keep plateaus at bay by increasing your BMR.

REMEMBER THAT CHANGE NEVER STOPS.

Our bodies and lives are in a constant state of change. Marriages, divorces, job transfers, pregnancies, injuries, illnesses, and hormonal transitions are just some of the many things that keep us in flux. Because of this, as you reach your initial goals, you may decide that you want even greater results. Or unexpected things might happen in your life that make you reevaluate your original benchmarks and downshift your expectations. Just know that with every change that comes into your life, you have the power to be in control of the way you handle that change.

Dealing with Obstacles

To prepare yourself for the barriers to brain health and weight loss, take time to think about the challenges you will face and how you will handle them. Use the chart below to write down your obstacles and plans to deal with them.

My Obstacles to Brain Health and Weight Loss	How I Will Deal with These Obstacles
_____	_____
_____	_____
_____	_____
_____	_____
_____	_____

The Amen Solution All-Stars: Cam Cleeland

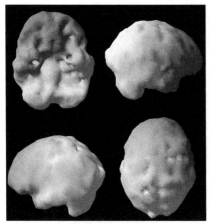
Cam's brain—before

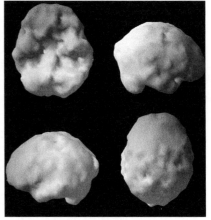
Cam's brain—after

At thirty-four, Cam Cleeland is one of our younger retired NFL players. He played football at a very high level in high school, in college at the University of Washington, and eight years in the pros as a tight end with the New Orleans Saints, New England Patriots, and St. Louis Rams. At age thirty-four, he volunteered for our study because he was struggling with problems of depression, irritability, low tolerance for frustration, high stress, obsessive thinking, and memory problems.

While playing football in college, he had a concussion and was unconscious for eighteen hours. He was diagnosed with a total of eight concussions—three in college and five in the pros. He said his "bell was rung" every week.

Once, in his rookie year while playing for Mike Ditka in New Orleans, he was involved in a hazing incident during which other players whacked him on the head with socks filled with coins (not a sign of intelligent life). Cam suffered a concussion and vision problems after the incident. Cam said that the NFL changed its position on hazing after the incident.

Cam's evaluation showed clear evidence of depression, brain trauma, and cognitive dysfunction. His SPECT scan showed left-sided brain damage (he said he was hit in the left eye during the hazing incident and that he felt better on blocks when he led with the left side of his head). His Microcog (a test of neuropsychological function) showed significant decreases in general cognitive functioning, information processing speed, attention, memory, and spatial processing.

As part of our study, we put Cam on our brain rehabilitation program, which included fish oil (Omega-3 Power), a great multiple vitamin (NeuroVite), and our Brain & Memory Power Boost.

Eight months later we reassessed Cam, using the same protocol as before. He reported he felt much better and noticed significant improvements in his attention, mental clarity, memory, mood, motivation, and anxiety level. He felt his anger was under greater control and he was getting along better with his small children.

His SPECT scan showed dramatic improvement in the areas of his temporal lobes (memory and mood stability), prefrontal cortex (attention and judgment), and cerebellum (processing speed). His Microcog showed dramatic improvement as well (see the following table).

He feels the difference and is excited to do everything he can to change his brain and change his life. You see, changing your brain can make you smarter and happier! It also made him thinner—Cam has lost 25 pounds since starting the program.

CAM CLEELAND'S MICROCOG RESULTS

	Before	*After*	*%Change*
General cognitive functioning	13	39	200%+
Information processing speed	12	30	150%+
Information processing accuracy	27	55	100%+
Attention	34	70	100%+
Memory	30	77	>150%+
Spatial processing	5	77	>1,400%+

The numbers are Cam's percentile rankings, comparing him with other people his age and education level. For example, the 5 percent in Spatial Processing means 95 percent of people his age and education scored better than Cam.

APPENDIX A

THE AMEN SOLUTION
MASTER QUESTIONNAIRE

THE AMEN SOLUTION Questionnaire is a great place to start helping you evaluate your own individual brain. For many years, I realized that not everyone is able to get a brain scan to check on the health of his or her brain. So, in order to bring the life-changing information to as many people as possible, I developed this questionnaire to help predict the areas of strengths and vulnerabilities of the brain.

A word of caution is in order. Self-report questionnaires have advantages and limitations. They are quick and easy to score. On the other hand, people filling them out may portray themselves in a way they want to be perceived, resulting in self-report bias. For example, some people exaggerate and mark all of the symptoms as frequent, in essence saying, "I'm glad to have a problem so that I can get help or have an excuse for the troubles I have." Others are in denial. They do not want to see any personal flaws and they do not check any symptoms as significant, in essence saying, "I'm okay. There's nothing wrong with me. Leave me alone." Not all self-report bias is intentional. People may genuinely have difficulty recognizing and expressing how they feel. Sometimes family members or friends are better at evaluating a loved one's level of functioning than a person evaluating him- or herself.

Questionnaires of any sort should never be used as the only assessment tool. Use this one as a catalyst to help you think, ask better questions, and get more evaluation if needed. Always discuss any recommendations with your personal physician or health care provider, especially if you are taking any medications, such as for your heart, asthma, diabetes, blood thinners, blood pressure, or for anxiety, depression, or pain.

THE AMEN SOLUTION
Master Questionnaire
Copyright © 2011 Daniel Amen, M.D.

Please rate yourself on each of the symptoms listed below using the following scale. If possible, to give yourself the most complete picture, have another person who knows you well (such as a spouse, lover, or parent) rate you as well. List the other person: _____

0	1	2	3	4	NA
Never	Rarely	Occasionally	Frequently	Very Frequently	Not Applicable/ known

Other Self

1. Trouble sustaining attention
2. Lacks attention to detail
3. Easily distracted
4. Procrastinate until I have to do something
5. Restless
6. Loses things
7. Difficulty expressing empathy for others
8. Blurts out answers, interrupts frequently
9. Impulsive (saying or doing things without thinking first)
10. Needs caffeine or nicotine in order to focus
11. Gets stuck on negative thoughts
12. Worries excessively
13. Tendency toward compulsive or addictive behaviors
14. Holds grudges
15. Upset when things do not go your way
16. Upset when things are out of place
17. Tendency to be oppositional or argumentative
18. Dislikes change
19. Needing to have things done a certain way or you become very upset

____ ____ 20. Trouble seeing options in situations

____ ____ 21. Feeling sad

____ ____ 22. Being negative

____ ____ 23. Feeling dissatisfied

____ ____ 24. Feeling bored

____ ____ 25. Low energy

____ ____ 26. Decreased interest in things that are usually fun or pleasurable

____ ____ 27. Feelings of hopelessness, helplessness, worthlessness, or guilt

____ ____ 28. Crying spells

____ ____ 29. Chronic low self-esteem

____ ____ 30. Social isolation

____ ____ 31. Feelings of nervousness and anxiety

____ ____ 32. Feelings of panic

____ ____ 33. Symptoms of heightened muscle tension, such as headaches or sore muscles

____ ____ 34. Tendency to predict the worst

____ ____ 35. Avoid conflict

____ ____ 36. Excessive fear of being judged or scrutinized by others

____ ____ 37. Excessive motivation, trouble stopping work

____ ____ 38. Lacks confidence in their abilities

____ ____ 39. Always watching for something bad to happen

____ ____ 40. Easily startled

____ ____ 41. Temper problems

____ ____ 42. Short fuse

____ ____ 43. Irritability tends to build, then explodes, then recedes, often tired after a rage

____ ____ 44. Unstable or unpredictable moods

____ ____ 45. Misinterprets comments as negative when they are not

____ ____ 46. Déjà vu (feelings of being somewhere you have never been)

____ ____ 47. Often feel as though others are watching you or out to hurt you

____ ____ 48. Dark or violent thoughts, that may come out of the blue

____ ____ 49. Trouble finding the right word to say

____ ____ 50. Headaches or abdominal pain of uncertain origin

____ ____ 51. Snores loudly or others complain about your snoring

____ ____ 52. Other say you stop breathing when you sleep

____ ____ 53. Feel fatigued or tired during the day

___ ___ 54. Agitated, easily upset, nervous when meals are missed

___ ___ 55. Get lightheaded if meals are missed

___ ___ 56. Eating relieves fatigue

___ ___ 57. Diet is poor and tends to be haphazard

___ ___ 58. Do not exercise

___ ___ 59. Put myself at risk for brain injuries, by doing such things as not wearing my seat belt, drinking and driving, engaging in high risk sports, etc.

___ ___ 60. Live under daily or chronic stress, in my home or work life

___ ___ 61. Thoughts tend to be negative, worried, or angry

___ ___ 62. Problems getting at least six to seven hours of sleep a night

___ ___ 63. Smoke or am exposed to secondhand smoke

___ ___ 64. Drink or consume more than two cups of coffee, tea, or dark sodas a day

___ ___ 65. Use aspartame and/or MSG

___ ___ 66. Spends time around environmental toxins, such as paint fumes, hair or nail salon fumes, or pesticides

___ ___ 67. Spend more than one hour a day watching TV

___ ___ 68. Spend more than one hour a day playing video games

___ ___ 69. Outside of work time, spend more than one hour a day on the computer

___ ___ 70. Consume more than three normal-size drinks of alcohol a week

___ ___ 71. Struggle with being overweight and/or wish to lose weight

THE AMEN SOLUTION
MASTER QUESTIONNAIRE

ANSWER KEY

Place the number of questions you, or a significant other, answered 3 or 4 in the space provided.

_____ 1–10 Prefrontal cortex problems (read more in chapter 4).

_____ 11–20 Anterior cingulate gyrus problems (read more in chapter 4).

_____ 21–30 Deep limbic system problems (read more in chapter 4).

_____ 31–40 Basal ganglia problems (read more in chapter 4).

_____ 41–50 Temporal lobe problems (read more in chapter 4).

For the five brain systems above, find below the likelihood that a problem exists. If there is a potential problem, see the corresponding section of the book.

5 questions = Highly probable
3 questions = Probable
2 questions = May be possible

_____ 51–53 Sleep apnea. If you answered one or more of these questions with a score of 3 or 4, you may have sleep apnea. Sleep apnea occurs when people stop breathing multiple times during the night. It causes significant oxygen deprivation for the brain and people often feel tired and depressed. This condition is best evaluated by a sleep study in a specialized sleep laboratory. Treating sleep apnea often makes a positive difference in mood and energy. If you suspect a problem talk to your physician.

_____ 54–56 Hypoglycemia. If you answered three or more questions with a score of 3 or 4, low blood sugar states should be evaluated by your physician. Low blood sugar or hypoglycemia can cause symptoms of anxiety and lethargy. Eating four to five small meals a day, as well as eliminating most of the simple sugars in your diet (such as sugar, bread, pasta, potatoes, and rice) can be very helpful to balance your mood and anxiety levels.

_____ 57–70 Bad brain habit questions. For these questions, add up your total score, not just the ones you answered 3 or 4.

If you score between 0 and 6, odds are you have very good brain habits. Congratulations!

If you score between 7 and 12, odds are you are doing well, but you can work to be better.

If you score between 13 and 20, your brain habits are not good and you are prematurely aging your brain. A better brain awaits you.

If you score more than 20, you have poor brain habits and it is time to be concerned. A brain makeover may just change your life!

_____ 71. Overweight issues. If you scored 3 or 4 on this question, look on page 276 to help you determine if you have a brain type associated with overeating. Not everyone has a type. If you don't have a type, use all of the other ideas in *The Amen Solution* to get control of your health.

THE AMEN SOLUTION
KNOW YOUR BRAIN TYPE

TYPE 1: THE COMPULSIVE OVEREATER

- If you answered yes to question 71
- Plus a score of 3 or more on five questions from 11 to 20, you are likely to have the compulsive overeating type of weight issue.
- *See chapter 4 for information and suggestions for helpful interventions.*

TYPE 2: THE IMPULSIVE OVEREATER

- If you answered yes to question 71
- Plus a score of 3 or more on five questions from 1 to 10, you are likely to have the impulsive overeating type of weight issue.
- *See chapter 4 for information and suggestions for helpful interventions.*

TYPE 3: THE IMPULSIVE-COMPULSIVE OVEREATER

- If you answered yes to question 71
- Plus a score of 3 or more on five questions from both 1 to 10 and 11 to 20, you are likely to have the impulsive-compulsive overeating type of weight issue.
- *See chapter 4 for information and suggestions for helpful interventions.*

TYPE 4: THE SAD OR EMOTIONAL OVEREATER

- If you answered yes to question 71
- Plus a score of 3 or more on five questions from 21 to 30, you are likely to have the sad or emotional overeating type of weight issue.
- *See chapter 4 for information and suggestions for helpful interventions.*

TYPE 5: THE ANXIOUS OVEREATER

- If you answered yes to question 71
- Plus a score of 3 or more on five questions from 31 to 40, you are likely to have the anxious overeating type of weight issue.
- *See chapter 4 for information and suggestions for helpful interventions*

Chapter 4 has instructions on what to do if you have more than one type.

APPENDIX B
TWO HUNDRED WAYS TO
LEAVE YOUR BLUBBER BEHIND

Here are two hundred easy ways to slash calories, burn calories, boost self-control, and slim down.

1. Stop thinking that breakfast equals baked goods. Scramble two egg whites with 3 ounces chopped chicken breast and ½ cup spinach instead of eating a 350-calorie whole-wheat sesame bagel to cut nearly 160 calories and boost your focus.

2. Try 1 cup cooked quinoa with berries instead of your favorite sweetened cereal to boost protein content and keep you feeling full longer. You'll eat fewer calories throughout the day.

3. Ditch the chocolate frosted doughnuts (540 calories for two) and get smart by making veggies a part of your breakfast. Put spinach, celery, and broccoli in a blender with 1 scoop vanilla whey protein powder to cut nearly 400 calories.

4. Use 2 tablespoons fruit-only, no-sugar-added jams instead of regular jam for bagels or toast and save about 20 calories. This also helps to get rid of the extra sugar.

5. Replace two slices of regular bacon (80 calories) at breakfast with two slices of fat-free turkey bacon (40 calories) to cut 40 calories.

6. Indulge in modified French toast. Use ½ cup unsweetened almond milk and 2 egg whites instead of whole milk and eggs to trim about 150 calories. Use sprouted grain bread instead of white bread to boost fiber and nutrient content.

7. If you love pancakes, use oat flour or brown rice flour and ditch the syrup, which costs 104 calories for two tablespoons. Top with ½ cup of sliced fresh strawberries and ½ cup of blueberries instead and save at least 40 calories.

8. Eat breakfast every day. People who skip breakfast are four times more likely to be fat than people who don't skip breakfast! The National Weight Control Registry, which includes people who have maintained at least a 30-pound weight loss for at least one year, reports that 78 percent of its members eat breakfast every day.

9. Don't reach for the all-American breakfast special (two slices of bacon, two fried eggs, and two pancakes with butter and syrup), which can add up to more than 800 calories in some restaurants. Rather a 200- to 300-calorie protein-blueberry shake is a good brain healthy way to start the day.

10. Top your steel-cut oatmeal with 1 cup unsweetened almond milk instead of whole milk to save 110 calories.

11. When you scramble or fry eggs, use cooking spray, which usually costs less than 10 calories per one second spray, rather than butter or margarine at 100 calories per tablespoon to save 90 calories or more.

12. Eat two poached eggs instead of fried eggs and save about 100 calories.

13. Try my favorite butter substitute: Earth Balance Natural Buttery Spread with Olive Oil. It has no trans fats, less than half the saturated fat of real butter, and 20 fewer calories per serving compared with real butter or margarine.

14. Eat only the egg white and toss away the yolk to trim about 60 calories.

15. Substitute 1% or fat-free cottage cheese for 2% and save at least 60 calories per cup.

16. Skip the cheese and Italian sausage in your omelet and add spinach, mushrooms, tomatoes, or bell peppers instead and trim more than 300 calories.

17. Replace 1 tablespoon regular mayo (90 calories) on your turkey sandwich with 1 tablespoon of reduced-fat mayo to cut 40 calories. Or save about 80 calories with 1 tablespoon of fat-free mayo.

18. Add more vegetables, such as cucumbers, lettuce, tomato, and onions to a sandwich instead of extra meat or cheese and save about 200 calories.

19. Accompany a sandwich with salad or fruit instead of chips or French fries and cut anywhere from 150 to more than 500 calories depending on serving size.

20. Choose vegetable-based broth soups rather than cream- or meat-based soups. With one famous soup brand, you'll save at least 100 calories per cup this way.

21. Stop putting butter, margarine, or mayonnaise on your sandwiches. Use mustard instead and save up to 95 calories per tablespoon.

22. Use water-packed tuna instead of tuna packed in oil. A 5-ounce can of tuna in oil costs 220 calories whereas the water-packed tuna is only 100 calories.

23. Prepare tuna with nonfat mayonnaise instead of regular mayonnaise to trim 80 calories from your sandwich.

24. Skip the slice of cheese on your sandwich to save about 100 calories.

25. Say no to the free chips and soda with your deli sandwich to trim about 250 calories from your meal.

26. Use a 6-inch or 8-inch taco-size sprouted grain flourless or brown rice tortilla instead of a 10-inch burrito-size flour tortilla and save 40–100 calories.

27. Switch to a 6-inch corn tortilla instead of a 10-inch flour tortilla and save 165 calories.

28. Steam veggies instead of sautéing them in 2 tablespoons butter or oil and cut 200 calories.

29. Switch to four boiled shrimp instead of 4 ounces of sirloin steak on shish kebabs to trim more than 100 calories.

30. Broil or bake foods instead of frying them and cut hundreds of calories.

31. Try lemon juice to flavor vegetables instead of oil or butter and save about 100 calories per tablespoon.

32. Change your thinking. Think of vegetables as your "main dish" rather than your "side dish." You'll eat fewer calories that way.

33. Modify recipes to reduce the amount of fat and calories. For example, when making chili, load it up with shredded vegetables, such as carrots, zucchini, and spinach and use just a small amount of ground white meat turkey instead of beef. You'll cut a couple hundred calories per serving.

34. Use 95 percent extra-lean ground beef rather than 70 percent ground beef to cut more than 100 calories per 4-ounce serving.

35. Eat sweet potatoes, which contain cellulose and hemicelluloses, insoluble fibers that help you feel full faster so you eat less.

36. Using fresh herbs and garlic instead of one tablespoon of butter or oil adds a lot of flavor and saves about 100 calories.

37. Brown and basmati rice are a good carbohydrate fix because as little as a half cup is very filling and has a higher nutritional value than white rice as well as a lower glycemic index factor so you get more bang for your buck.

38. Mix ½ cup pinto beans with ½ cup brown rice to create a complete protein and a low-calorie alternative to meat. Adding fresh herbs, garlic, and salsa or low-salt Italian diced tomatoes is delicious and adds up to less than 250 calories.

39. Swap quinoa for white rice. Quinoa is a complete protein and contains more protein than any other grain with 9 grams per 1 cup of cooked quinoa. It is much lower on the glycemic index than white rice, which helps you avoid a spike in blood sugar. This can improve self-control and reduce the calories you consume for the rest of the day.

40. Trim the fat from all meat and avoid eating the skin on poultry to cut about 50 calories.

41. Squeeze lemon juice on fish instead of 2 tablespoons of tartar sauce and save 70 calories.

42. Make 99 percent fat-free white-meat turkey meatballs instead of 95 percent extra lean beef meatballs to save about 65 calories per serving.

43. Use grilled portobello mushrooms instead of 95 percent extra-lean beef in your burger and save about 140 calories.

44. Go bunless. Have your burger on a bed of lettuce instead of a bun and lop off 150 calories or more.

45. At Chinese restaurants, just say no to the fried crunchy noodles they put on wonton soup and save about 150 calories.

46. Make your own salad dressings, such as balsamic vinegar with a little fresh garlic. In restaurants, use straight balsamic vinegar or lemon juice to cut 100 calories per tablespoon compared with other dressings.

47. Limit salad toppings. A big salad might seem healthy, but all those goodies on top can make it more calorie-laden than lasagna or fettuccine Al-

fredo. Cheese crumbles, caramelized nuts, bacon, avocado, dried fruit, croutons, and creamy dressings can add lots of calories. Save 500 or more calories by having just one topping, adding flavorful but lower-cal veggies (roasted bell peppers, grilled onions, or mushrooms), and using half the dressing.

48. Vinegar and citrus fruits are great substitutes for cream sauces on just about anything, and they can cut hundreds of calories.

49. Spaghetti squash and shredded zucchini are excellent substitutes for pasta and taste like whatever you add to it. You save almost 200 calories per cup.

50. "Clean your plate" is one of the worst habits we are taught. Stop eating when you feel full and save the rest for leftovers. This one habit can cut hundreds of calories from your daily intake.

51. To learn how to stop cleaning your plate, make it a practice to leave two or three bites of food on your plate at every meal. The few bites won't add up to that many calories but learning not to devour everything a restaurant or dinner host serves you can save hundreds of calories on those occasions.

52. The best way to limit your calories is to cook at home where you can control the amount of food on your plate. This can slash hundreds or even more than 1,000 calories in some cases.

53. If you must have a high-calorie food at a meal, eat the more nutritious, low-calorie foods on your plate first. Then you likely won't eat as much of the high-calorie food.

54. Substitute lower-calorie fish like halibut for steak to trim 80 or more calories per serving.

55. Swap ½ cup steamed brown rice for ½ cup fried rice and save about 100 calories.

56. If you can't live without fries (427 calories for a medium order), skip the frying and make baked sweet potato fries, which are about 100 calories per serving. You save almost 300 calories and you gain loads of brain healthy nutrients.

57. Say no to fried and breaded chicken and opt for grilled or baked chicken instead to cut at least 100 calories per serving.

58. Less is more when it comes to brain healthy preparation. Eat vegetables raw without any oil, butter, or cream sauces to save hundreds of calories.

59. With pasta, use marinara sauce instead of Alfredo sauce to save 260 calories per cup or instead of pesto sauce to cut 440 calories per cup.

60. Put less food on your plate than you think you need. You can always go back to the kitchen for more if you are still hungry, but you might find that you feel full with less food. You can knock off hundreds of calories with this trick.

61. Never order salad with the dressing already tossed. Get it on the side, so you are in control of how much you eat, and dip your fork in it before you grab the salad mix. You will likely cut the calories from the dressing in half—or even more—and miss none of the taste. Considering how much dressing restaurants pour on, this could easily be several hundred calories.

62. When you use olive oil and vinegar on salad, liberally put the vinegar on first, then add just a few drops of olive oil. You will likely cut more than 100 calories from your meal.

63. Steam broccoli and asparagus instead of cooking in 2 tablespoons butter to save 200 calories.

64. Eat more veggies. Researchers at Tufts University found that the more vegetables people eat, the thinner they are.

65. Change the proportion of ingredients so that the same amount of food has more vegetables or fruits, which are filling and low in calories. For example, instead of 1 cup brown rice, 4 ounces 95 percent extra-lean ground beef, ½ cup of shredded low-fat cheddar cheese, and 1/4 cup red bell peppers (total of about 550 calories), use 2 cups red bell peppers, ½ cup rice, 3 ounces ground beef, and ¼ cup cheese and save about 180 calories.

66. Switch to plain, unsweetened yogurt and add your own fruit. You can get the health benefits from yogurt and eliminate about 50 calories per 6-ounce serving and unwanted sugar.

67. Bring low-calorie snacks to school or work. I like raw broccoli, cauliflower, carrots, snap peas, celery, and red bell peppers. I may also bring a measured portion of almond butter or mashed avocado with garlic powder as a dip. It is important not to let yourself get hungry.

68. Eat a medium-sized apple shortly after meals. The fiber will help you continue to feel full hours later so you don't raid the refrigerator, which can add up to hundreds of unwanted calories.

69. Dip carrots, red bell peppers, or celery instead of tortilla chips into your favorite salsa, guacamole, or hummus to save about 140 calories.

70. When you make air-popped popcorn, put half of it away to eat for another time. If you pop 6 cups, put 3 cups away to shave 90 calories.

71. For people who have a sweet tooth like me, eat a small portion of something sweet, like blueberries (20 calories for ¼ cup) or dark chocolate (about 20 calories for one piece of Hershey's Kisses dark chocolate), so that you can have something satisfying without feeling like you are depriving yourself.

72. Choose crunchy things. Scientists say the more you chew, the longer it takes to eat and the more time your body has to realize that it is full. Snacks that offer a big crunch include carrots, apples, snap peas, and nuts (processed carbohydrates like sugar cereals and candy don't count). They keep your mouth busy longer so you don't inhale your food like a vacuum cleaner.

73. Read the fine print. To get the real scoop on a snack, check out the back of the box. When you see a list of hard-to-pronounce ingredients, there is a greater chance something artificial is mixed in that is not necessarily waistline-friendly. A shorter list usually indicates a more nutritious and slimming pick.

74. At the movies, bring 3 cups popcorn that you air-popped at home instead of getting the large tub at the concession stand and save more than 1,500 calories at some theaters.

75. If you're buying canned fruit cocktail, you can save more than 100 calories per cup by choosing fruit packed in water rather than heavy syrup.

76. Avoid the vending machine by packing your own healthful snacks to bring to work. For example, consider vegetable sticks, fresh fruit, or low-fat or nonfat yogurt without added sugars. Compared with a candy bar from the vending machine, you can save up to 200 calories if you eat the raw veggies.

77. Tree nuts can be a very healthy snack, as long as you don't eat too many of them. One ounce (about one handful) of dry-roasted mixed nuts has about 175 calories. Take one handful and seal the bag rather than nibbling straight from the bag to keep the calorie count down.

78. Choose 1 cup red grapes instead of 1 cup raisins to save about 450 calories.

79. Skip the dried fruit with added sugar and eat a piece of fresh fruit to cut up to several hundred calories.

80. When your dinner hosts serve dessert, excuse yourself and go for a walk. By skipping dessert, you can easily cut hundreds of calories.

81. Eat a low-sugar protein bar in the afternoon instead of a candy bar. The calorie counts may be similar but the protein will help regulate your blood sugar and help your self-control later in the evening while the candy bar will lead to a sugar crash and a greater likelihood of overeating at night.

82. Instead of spending 400-plus calories on a slice of chocolate cheese-cake, have a single piece of dark chocolate after dinner and save more than 350 calories. A little bit of dark chocolate a day has healthy benefits, including increasing blood flow to the brain and decreasing blood pressure, but make sure you count the calories.

83. Have frozen blueberries with 1 cup Greek-style nonfat yogurt and a little stevia—delicious and only about 150 calories—instead of 1 cup rich ice cream at 540 calories.

84. Frozen red grapes make a great dessert and are about 450 fewer calories per cup than ice cream.

85. Instead of store-bought sorbet, make your own by putting fruit in the blender and then pouring into Popsicle trays. You'll save about 100 calories per serving.

86. For dessert, forget the slice of apple pie (500 calories or more!) from your favorite restaurant and have a small baked apple sprinkled with cinnamon and nutmeg. It's delicious and slashes more than 400 calories.

87. Eat a banana with 1 tablespoon almond butter (about 200 calories) rather than a slice of banana cream pie with whipped cream to cut more than 350 calories.

88. Satisfy sweet-tooth cravings with a cup of hot or iced fruity tea with a little stevia and save up to several hundred calories.

89. Fluff up your food. In one study from Penn State, twenty-eight men drank one of three different kinds of milkshakes before lunch. All three milkshakes had the same ingredients, but some were blended longer to add air and volume. The men who drank the "airy" shakes ate 12 percent fewer calories at lunch. And they did not make up for it by eating more at dinner, meaning they kept those calories off. So if you are going to have a protein shake for dessert or for breakfast like I do, blend it longer to add more air.

90. Switch to water first thing in the morning instead of fruit juice. Fruit juice is high in sugar and just 1 cup orange juice costs 112 calories.

91. Instead of drinking fruit juice, eat a piece of fruit. The fruit has fiber, which slows the absorption of the natural sugars to keep your blood sugar

levels from spiking. Eating one medium orange instead of a 12-ounce glass of orange juice can cut 80 calories.

92. Stop drinking soda. Regular sodas are filled with sugar and caffeine and cost 150 calories each. The artificial sweeteners from diet sodas may be calorie-free, but they are harmful to your health. Plus, because they are up to six hundred times sweeter than sugar, they may activate the appetite centers of the brain making you crave even more food. So the 150 calories you saved by drinking the diet soda may be spent later that day.

93. Replace sodas with real fruit-flavored water, just like you are at the spa. My favorite drink is water with lemon juice and a little lemon-flavored stevia, a healthier natural sweetener. It has no calories and it tastes like lemonade. You can do it with oranges, limes, watermelon, and so on. This is an easy way to dramatically increase your water intake and save 150 calories per glass.

94. Don't let the sports drinks and vitamin waters fake you out. The truth is most are just sweetened water that will cost more than 100 calories for 12 ounces.

95. If you can't kick your sports drink habit, pour half of the bottle into a glass and mix with an equal amount of water and fill up the bottle with water also to cut the calories and sugar in half.

96. Don't let beverage labels pull a fast one on you. If it is not water, unsweetened almond milk, decaf coffee, or unsweetened tea, it is dessert.

97. Limit alcohol, especially mixed drinks, which can have an outrageous number of calories. For example, one margarita can have as many as 700 calories! Plus, the alcohol decreases prefrontal cortex function, which means your judgment will be impaired, making you more likely to eat more high-fat, high-sugar, high-calorie foods.

98. Going from one glass of wine every night at dinner to one glass per week can trim about 600 calories per week.

99. If you're going to drink, skip the Long Island iced tea (upwards of 500 calories) and go for one glass of white wine (less than 100 calories) to save more than 400 calories.

100. Limit fat storage by drinking green tea, which contains the antioxidant epigallocatechin gallate (EGCG), shown to boost metabolic rate. In a recent three-month study, participants who took green tea extract lost 4.6 percent of their body weight without changing their diet. To get the benefit,

drink at least three cups a day. My favorite is Tropical Acai Berry Green Tea by Celestial Seasonings.

101. Before meals, drink fiber—such as Citrucel, Metamucil, or MiraLAX (with lots of water)—because it fills the belly, so there is less room for food.

102. When you get hungry, first drink a full glass of water and then if you are still hungry, eat. Many people confuse being dehydrated with being hungry.

103. Drink ice-cold water. Your body burns a few calories warming up the water to body temperature. Drinking an 8-ounce glass of ice cold water burns about 8 calories. Granted, it's not much, but calories are calories.

104. Use almond milk instead of cow's milk. Blue Diamond unsweetened almond milk contains only 40 calories for 8 ounces. Their unsweetened chocolate almond milk contains only 45 calories and is delicious. I actually like almond milk better than cow's milk.

105. Another milk alternative is unsweetened rice milk. It will cut more than 100 calories per cup.

106. Stop using half-and-half in your coffee or tea. Switch to unsweetened almond milk to cut more than 17 calories per tablespoon.

107. Sprinkle cinnamon or nutmeg in your coffee rather than using flavored syrups, which can cost 20 calories per squirt at your favorite coffeehouse.

108. Using stevia is a great no-calorie way to sweeten drinks like coffee and tea and most foods. Stevia is 100 percent natural, and it has no effect on blood sugar. Compared with 11 calories per packet of sugar, the savings add up.

109. Avoid high-calorie coffee drinks. You can cut more than 600 calories by switching from some fancy coffee drinks to a plain drip (decaf preferably) coffee with a little unsweetened almond milk and stevia.

110. Split meals with your spouse or friends when you eat out to cut calories by half.

111. If you are eating out by yourself, have your server put half your meal in a "to go" bag before serving you. That way, you won't be tempted to clean your plate.

112. In restaurants, ask if you can substitute a broth-based soup for French fries or chips as a side dish so you can save well over 100 calories.

113. Barbara Rolls, a nutrition researcher at Pennsylvania State University and author of *The Volumetrics Eating Plan: Techniques and Recipes for Feeling Full on Fewer Calories,* conducted a study that found that people who ate 1 cup low-calorie vegetable broth before lunch reduced their total calorie intake by 20 percent.

114. Don't make a lot of different dishes for your meals. Research shows that the more choices you have the more you typically eat.

115. After hosting family gatherings, immediately give away or discard any foods that are not on your everyday diet. If the food is perfectly good, take it to your local food bank or share it with a neighbor.

116. Eat a snack or a light meal before you go to a party so you won't be hungry when faced with high-calorie hors d'oeuvres.

117. Skip the bread they serve before meals in restaurants. At one popular restaurant, a single breadstick adds 150 calories to your meal. And who can stop at just one?

118. Eating at a Chinese restaurant? Use chopsticks. It slows down consumption so you feel full faster and eat less.

119. Don't order appetizers before your entrée—unless it's a broth-based soup.

120. Tell your waiter "No croutons" on your salad. One cup of the crunchy salad toppers can cost more than 185 calories.

121. Be picky. If you don't *love* something that's on your plate, don't eat it. You can save hundreds of calories this way.

122. Use your brain to always think "high-quality calories in." Focus on calorie-restricted and optimally nutritious foods when you are deciding what to eat.

123. Stay away from "anti-nutrition" foods—such as trans fats, negative calories, or potentially harmful food additives—even if they are low in calories. Ultimately, they can spike your appetite and make you eat even more.

124. Don't add sugar to anything. A single teaspoon of the sweet stuff adds 16 calories.

125. Don't think you are doing yourself a favor by using brown sugar, raw sugar, turbinado sugar, agave syrup, or honey. They all contain calories you don't need.

126. Beware of fat-free products. Fat-free does not mean calorie-free. Check the nutrition label before you indulge.

127. One of the best ways to cut calories is to write down and measure everything you eat until you are confident that you really know how many calories you put into your body every day. Studies show that most people tend to underestimate the number of calories in a meal, but overweight individuals have a greater amount of portion distortion. Seeing is believing.

128. Serve your food on smaller plates, which will help to shrink your serving sizes. Turn in your 12-inch plate for a 10-inch version to cut 20 to 25 percent of your calories. You can thank Brian Wansink, author of *Mindless Eating,* and his team of researchers at the Cornell University Food and Brand Lab for the research behind this tip as well as the following five tips.

129. Going to a buffet? Sit at least sixteen feet away from and don't face the buffet table. Researchers at the Cornell University Food and Brand Lab found that fatter diners tend to sit closer to the buffet and return more often for more helpings than slimmer people.

130. Use smaller bowls when eating cereal, yogurt, or soup. Research shows that the bigger your bowl, the more you will eat.

131. Go small with serving utensils too. It isn't just the size of the plates and bowls you eat from that influence your calorie intake, it is also the size of the serving spoons you use. Bigger spoons equal bigger portions.

132. Don't put the serving bowls and platters on the table. That makes it too easy to take seconds . . . and thirds. Leave the serving dishes in the kitchen to cut calories.

133. Say no to big dinner parties with lots of guests. You tend to eat more when there are more than seven people at the table.

134. In a restaurant, always ask how your meal is prepared and request "no butter," "no cheese," and so on. You can cut hundreds of calories with this simple trick.

135. Substitute lower-fat meats—such as turkey, chicken, or lean pork—for higher-fat, higher-calorie alternatives. For example, choosing a chicken breast instead of prime rib can trim more than 300 calories per serving.

136. Lean on low-density foods to help you feel fuller faster. Low-density foods typically contain more water so you can eat larger portions yet fewer calories. High-density foods, on the other hand, pack lots of calories in very small portions. Be a value spender and go for the low-density variety. For ex-

ample, for the same number of calories, you could either eat 1 ounce French fries or 9 ounces fresh strawberries.

137. Chew each bite 20 times. One study found that diners with higher body mass indexes (BMIs) chewed each bite only twelve times compared with an average of fifteen times for healthy-weight people. Try to savor the food. In essence, you are performing a mindful meditation when you eat. This also makes your food taste sweeter. Saliva has an enzyme called amylase that breaks down simple carbohydrates, such as wheat or potatoes, into sugar.

138. Use all of your senses when you eat or drink. Pay attention to the favors, smells, textures, colors, and even the sounds they make when you consume them. This will help you eat more slowly, which can help you feel full on fewer calories.

139. Eat with your fork in your nondominant hand to reduce dexterity and slow down the shoveling of food into your mouth.

140. Put down your fork after each bite.

141. Cut down on the variety you eat, so that you actually know what is in your food. Gorillas tend to eat the same thing, over and over, and they are obviously strong and muscular. According to the National Zoo, here are the main ingredients of their diet: "The morning diet is generally made up of vegetables, which may include kale, celery, green beans, carrots, and sweet potato. Evening foods include more greens such as romaine, kale, cabbage, or dandelion along with the fruits and vegetables du jour. Bananas, apples, oranges, mango, grapes, melon, and papaya are often included. Onions, broccoli, turnips, white potatoes, squash, cucumbers, and beets are also included. Throughout the day, the gorillas are given additional forage items, such as popcorn, peanuts, or jungle mix. Browse (fresh tree trimmings) is given daily and includes bamboo, bradford pear, willow, mulberry, or maple."

142. Learn to eyeball servings. After you spend some time weighing food, learn about serving sizes. A 3-ounce serving of meat or poultry is about the size of a deck of cards, one serving of pasta or rice is the size of a tennis ball, a bread serving is the size of a CD case, and one serving of cheese is the size of four dice. See more suggested serving sizes in appendix C.

143. Eat at the table. Fifty-nine percent of young women eat on the go, a study in the *Journal of the American Dietetic Association* finds, and on-the-run eaters consume more total fat as well as more soda and fast food. The less

distracted and stressed you are when you dine, the more efficiently your body absorbs nutrients. Eat at the table and focus on your food, not the traffic.

144. Don't eat in front of the TV. In one study, people ate up to 44 percent more while watching TV compared with when they weren't in front of the boob tube.

145. For virtually no calories, adding spice to your meals can increase your metabolism. Different studies have shown that spicy foods can increase your metabolism by 8 to 20 percent for at least 30 minutes after eating. A little bit of cayenne pepper or cinnamon is all you need to add to your favorite recipes.

146. Eat veggies at every meal. When people eat vegetables with a meal, they consume a full 20 percent fewer calories overall while feeling satisfied, according to a study from the *American Journal of Clinical Nutrition.*

147. Increase your fiber intake. Eating fiber helps to prevent overeating because it makes you feel full. You will have an even greater feeling of fullness and higher energy levels throughout the day if you eat meals that are mostly made up of fiber, protein, and water. Fiber also slows down the digestion of foods you eat, keeping your blood sugar and energy levels in check and preventing you from getting hungry. Good sources of fiber are vegetables, fruits, nuts, beans, and some whole grain cereals. The amount of fiber in a food product is listed in the nutritional facts found on most food labels. Fiber takes so long to be digested by your body, a person eating 20–35 g fiber a day will burn an extra 150 calories a day or lose 16 extra pounds a year.

148. To get more fiber in your diet, ditch the white bread and replace it with whole wheat. A slice of white bread contains about ½ g fiber while whole wheat bread can be packed with 1.5 g to 7 g per slice. Check the labels to look for the highest fiber content.

149. Boost your fiber consumption by adding beans to soups and salads.

150. Make sure you eat healthy fats with every meal. It helps with satiety and serves to curb your appetite between meals. An Australian study showed that eating a meal with healthy fats, such as olive oil, significantly increased fat-burning rate five hours later, particularly in subjects with more abdominal fat.

151. Use a food scale to weigh and measure portion sizes and always measure the foods you tend to overeat.

152. Always measure and weigh the foods that you tend to overeat.

153. Make sure you have enough calcium in your diet. Researchers have linked calcium with lower production of the stress-hormone cortisol (remember cortisol switches the body into a fat-storing mode). According to several studies, people who increase their calcium intake lose more weight than people with low calcium levels. Sources of calcium include unsweetened yogurt and spinach.

154. Consistently reduce your meal sizes by just 10 percent. You won't even notice, and it will save an amazing number of calories.

155. Buy food in prepared-portioned sizes so you know exactly how many calories you are eating.

156. Get at least seven to eight hours of sleep at night. Getting fewer than that has been associated with eating more calories throughout the day and with eating more foods that can trigger cravings. One study in the *American Journal of Clinical Nutrition* found that people who got only five and a half hours of sleep ate 221 calories more than people who slept for eight and a half hours.

157. Liberally sprinkle cinnamon on your oatmeal in the morning to help regulate blood sugar levels. This will increase your self-control later in the day so you make better decisions and eat fewer calories.

158. Eat smaller, more frequent meals to keep blood sugar levels balanced and prevent overeating.

159. Eat with people who share your healthy lifestyle rather than eating with people who have bad eating habits. People tend to eat more when the people around them do so.

160. If you overeat one day, just get back on track the next day.

161. Learn to say no to friends and family members who offer you seconds or foods that don't fit into your brain healthy program. Simply saying no can trim hundreds of calories from your daily total.

162. Move more. James A. Levine, M.D., a researcher at the Mayo Clinic, has found that structured exercise isn't the only way to burn calories. Walking instead of taking the elevator, pacing while talking on the phone, and other everyday physical activities can burn an extra 500–1,000 calories per day. Levine calls this type of activity NEAT (non-exercise activity thermogenesis). I think it's pretty neat that you can burn so many calories so easily.

163. Pacing while talking on the phone for an hour can burn up to 115 calories more than sitting down.

164. Pump up your metabolism with strength training. The more muscle tissue you have the more calories you burn.

165. Some of the top calorie-burning activities are running at a fast pace, climbing stairs, and jumping rope. Notice that none of these requires expensive equipment or gym memberships.

166. Join a table tennis club to burn calories and boost your brain at the same time.

167. Spend thirty minutes gardening or mowing the lawn (not riding a lawn mower!) to burn 200 calories (based on a weight of 185 pounds).

168. One hour of heavy-duty housework can melt 400 calories (based on a weight of 185 pounds).

169. Spend half an hour washing your car to burn 200 calories (based on a weight of 185 pounds).

170. Moving to a new home can be a pain, but it sure burns a lot of calories. One hour of toting boxes can help you burn more than 600 calories (based on a weight of 185 pounds).

171. One hour of running around while playing with your kids can burn more than 400 calories (based on a weight of 185 pounds).

172. Shovel snow for just fifteen minutes to burn about 100 calories (based on a weight of 145 pounds).

173. Leave the car in the driveway and walk one hour to work or school at a quick clip to burn about 346 calories (based on a weight of 200 pounds). Double that if you walk back home too.

174. Just one hour of cleaning out the garage burns 329 calories (based on a weight of 145 pounds).

175. Spend thirty minutes scrubbing floors to burn 182 calories (based on a weight of 145 pounds).

176. Doing the laundry and folding clothes burns about 140 calories (based on a weight of 145 pounds).

177. Take half an hour to give your dog a bath and burn 156 pounds (based on a weight of 145 pounds).

178. Walk at a moderate pace while carrying your 12-pound baby and burn 230 calories in an hour (based on a weight of 145 pounds).

179. Pushing your toddler in a baby stroller burns about 165 calories per hour (based on a weight of 145 pounds).

180. Play guitar while standing for one hour, and you'll burn almost 200 calories (based on a weight of 145 pounds).

181. Rake leaves for half an hour to burn 165 calories (based on a weight of 185 pounds).

182. Join your company's softball team and burn more than 300 calories during an hour-long game (based on a weight of 145 pounds).

183. It has been estimated that the act of intercourse burns about 200 calories, the equivalent of running vigorously for thirty minutes. Most couples average about twenty-four minutes for lovemaking.

184. Strolling leisurely through the streets of a foreign city can burn about 135 calories (based on a weight of 145 pounds).

185. Go to the mall and try on clothes for an hour to burn about 135 calories (based on a weight of 145 pounds).

186. Go fish! Fishing can burn about 200 calories. Plus, you might catch something that's brain healthy and low-calorie to eat (based on a weight of 145 pounds).

187. Spend fifteen minutes juggling to burn about 65 calories and give your brain a great workout. Juggling has been found to enhance the white matter in the brain and improve connectivity between areas of the brain (based on a weight of 145 pounds).

188. Knitting for one hour burns about 100 calories and also boosts brainpower (based on a weight of 145 pounds).

189. Packing and unpacking your suitcases for fifteen minutes burns about 35 calories (based on a weight of 145 pounds)

190. Vary your workout to prevent boredom and to keep your body from getting too efficient at any one activity. Your body burns fewer calories when it gets more efficient.

191. Know your BMI and waist-to-height ratio. This will help you stop lying to yourself.

192. Know how many calories you need to eat to maintain your current weight. This will make you more aware of the number of calories you consume.

193. Optimize your vitamin D levels. Low levels of vitamin D have been linked to obesity.

194. Have your doctor check the health of your blood. People with low

blood counts can feel anxious and tired and may overeat as a way to medicate themselves.

195. Optimize thyroid levels. Low levels decrease overall brain activity and can impair self-control.

196. Optimize hormone levels. Low levels of testosterone and DHEA are associated with obesity.

197. Check your HgA1C level to test for diabetes. Having diabetes is associated with obesity.

198. Take the natural supplements recommended for your brain type. A balanced brain will boost your self-control and reduce the chances of overeating as a way to self-medicate.

199. Got cravings? Fight back with natural supplements that support craving control, such as alpha-lipoic acid, chromium, DL-phenylalanine, L-glutamine, and N-acetyl-cysteine.

200. Meditate to boost your prefrontal cortex and your self-control.

APPENDIX C

CALORIE COUNTS
(Alphabetical Order)

Food	Type	Serving	Calories
Apple	fresh	1 medium	72
Apple juice	unsweetened	1 cup	117
Applesauce	unsweetened	½ cup	50
Applesauce	sweetened	1 cup	100
Almonds	raw	10 whole	70
Almond butter	creamy, w/salt	1 tbsp.	100
Apricots	dried	1 cup, halves	313
Apricots	fresh	1 medium	17
Artichoke	cooked	1 medium	60
Artichoke hearts	cooked, boiled	½ cup	45
Asparagus	cooked	½ cup	20
Avocado	fresh	1 medium	322
Bacon	pan fried	1 slice	40
Bacon, turkey	extra lean	1 slice	20
Bagel	plain	1 large	280
Banana	fresh	1 medium	105
Beans	black, canned	½ cup	110
Beans	garbanzo, canned	½ cup	130
Beans	pinto, canned	½ cup	103
Beans	refried, canned	½ cup	140
Beef, ground	95% extra lean	4 oz.	185

Food	Type	Serving	Calories
Beef, ground	70% lean	4 oz.	305
Beer	light	12 oz.	100
Beer	regular	12 oz.	145
Beets	cooked	½ cup	37
Bell peppers	green, raw	1 cup, chopped	30
Bell peppers	red, raw	1 cup, chopped	46
Bell peppers	yellow, raw	1 cup, chopped	50
Blackberries	fresh	1 cup	62
Blueberries	fresh	1 cup	83
Bran flakes	cereal	¾ cup	96
Brazil nuts	roasted	1 oz.	190
Bread	white	1 slice	80
Bread	whole wheat	1 slice	69
Broccoli	cooked	1 spear	13
Broccoli	raw	1 spear	11
Brussels sprouts	cooked	1 cup	65
Bun, hamburger	white	1 bun	200
Bun, hamburger	whole wheat	1 bun	170
Bun, hot dog	whole wheat	1 bun	160
Butter, hard	salted	1 tbsp.	100
Cantaloupe	fresh	1 cup, diced	53
Carrots	cooked	1 cup	70
Carrots	raw	1 large	30
Cashews	dry roasted, with salt	1 oz.	163
Cashew butter	creamy, with salt	2 tbsp.	180
Catfish	cooked	3 oz.	128
Celery	raw	1 cup, diced	19
Celery	cooked	1 cup, diced	27
Cheese, cheddar	deli	1 slice	113
Cheese, cheddar	grated	1 cup	455
Cheese, cheddar	low-fat	1 slice	70
Cheese, ricotta	part skim milk	½ cup	171
Cheese, ricotta	whole milk	½ cup	216
Cheese, string	light	1 stick	60
Cheeseburger	regular condiments	1	359
Cherries	maraschino	1 medium	10
Cherries	fresh	½ cup	60
Chicken, dark meat	batter-fried with skin	½ chicken	830
Chicken breast	batter-fried with skin	4 oz.	294

Food	Type	Serving	Calories
Chicken breast	cooked, no skin	3 oz.	140
Chicken breast	deli meat	1 oz.	45
Chicken thigh	cooked, no skin	3 oz.	163
Chocolate, dark	73% cacao	1 oz.	50
Chocolate ice cream	regular	½ cup	143
Cod	cooked	3 oz.	88
Coffee	brewed	6 oz.	5
Cooking spray		1 second	<10
Corn	yellow, cooked	1 cup	177
Cottage cheese	nonfat	1 cup	104
Cottage cheese	1%	1 cup	163
Cottage cheese	2%	1 cup	226
Crab, blue	cooked	3 oz.	90
Craisins	dried	½ cup	184
Cranberries	fresh	1 cup	44
Cranberry juice	sweetened	1 cup	130
Cream cheese	fat-free	1 tbsp.	14
Cream cheese	regular	1 tbsp.	51
Croutons	seasoned	1 cup	186
Cucumbers	raw	1 medium	40
Dressing, Italian	Newman's Own	1 tbsp.	60
Dressing, ranch	Hidden Valley	1 tbsp.	100
Egg	hard-boiled	1 large	78
Egg	pan-fried	1 large	90
Egg white only	cooked	1 large	16
Feta cheese	regular	1 oz.	75
Filet mignon	lean, cooked	3 oz.	175
French fries	salted	medium order	427
Fruit cocktail	canned, heavy syrup	1 cup	181
Fruit cocktail	canned, light syrup	1 cup	138
Fruit cocktail	canned, water	1 cup	76
Garlic	fresh	1 clove	4
Granola	store-bought	½ cup	180
Grapefruit	fresh	½ fruit	52
Grapefruit juice	unsweetened	1 cup	96
Grapes	fresh, green	1 cup	58
Grapes	fresh, red	1 cup	60
Grape juice	unsweetened	1 cup	170
Green beans	cooked	1 cup	48

Food	Type	Serving	Calories
Ground beef	lean, cooked	3 oz.	164
Ground beef	regular, cooked	3 oz.	209
Ground turkey	lean, cooked	3 oz.	167
Halibut	cooked	3 oz.	120
Ham	deli meat	1 oz.	39
Hazelnuts	dry roasted	1 oz.	183
Herring, Atlantic	raw	4 oz.	179
Honey	100% pure	1 tbsp.	60
Honeydew	fresh	1 cup	60
Iceberg lettuce	fresh	1 cup, chopped	8
Ice cream	premium	½ cup	270
Ice cream, vanilla	regular	½ cup	145
Jam/jelly	strawberry	1 tbsp.	50
Jam/jelly	all-fruit spread	1 tbsp.	40
Jicama	raw	1 cup	49
Ketchup		1 tbsp.	15
Kiwi	fresh	1 medium	50
Lamb	cooked	3 oz.	269
Lemon juice	unsweetened	1 cup	61
Lemons	raw	1 slice	2
Lentils	boiled	½ cup	115
Lime juice	unsweetened	1 cup	62
Limes	fresh	1 lime	20
Lobster	cooked	3 oz.	110
Macadamia nuts	dry roasted	1 oz.	203
Mango	fresh	½ fruit	65
Margarine	hard	1 tbsp.	100
Mayonnaise	fat-free	1 tbsp.	11
Mayonnaise	light	1 tbsp.	50
Mayonnaise	regular	1 tbsp.	90
Milk	nonfat	1 cup	86
Milk	1%	1 cup	102
Milk	2%	1 cup	122
Milk	whole	1 cup	150
Milk	half-and-half	1 tbsp.	20
Milk, almond	chocolate flavor	1 cup	45
Milk, almond	unsweetened	1 cup	40
Mushrooms	cooked, no salt	1 cup	44
Mushrooms	raw	1 cup	15

Food	Type	Serving	Calories
Mushrooms, portobello	raw	1 cup	42
Mustard, yellow		1 tbsp.	3
Nectarine	fresh	1 medium	70
Nuts, mixed	dry roasted	1 oz.	175
Oatmeal	instant, cooked	1 cup	166
Oatmeal	rolled, dry	½ cup	150
Olive oil	extra-virgin	1 tbsp.	120
Olives	canned	1 tbsp.	10
Onion	raw	1 cup, diced	64
Orange	fresh	1 medium	85
Orange juice	unsweetened	1 cup	112
Papaya	fresh	½ medium	61
Parmesan cheese	grated	1 oz.	122
Peach	fresh	1 medium	38
Peanuts	dry roasted, with salt	1 oz.	166
Peanut butter	creamy, with salt	1 tbsp.	94
Pear	fresh	1 medium	96
Peas	boiled	½ cup	62
Pecans	raw	1 oz.	196
Pineapple	fresh	1 cup	75
Pineapple juice	unsweetened	1 cup	133
Pine nuts		1 oz.	191
Pistachios	dry roasted	1 oz.	161
Pizza, pepperoni	medium size	1 slice	215
Pizza, green peppers	medium size	1 slice	185
Plums	fresh	1 plum	30
Pomegranate	fresh	1 medium	105
Popcorn	air-popped	1 cup	30
Popcorn	oil-popped	1 cup	64
Pork chops	cooked	3 oz.	180
Pork tenderloin	cooked	3 oz.	140
Potato	brown, baked	1 medium	161
Potato	red, baked	1 medium	154
Potato chips	regular	20	150
Prime rib	cooked	3 oz.	355
Quinoa	cooked	½ cup	127
Raisins	seedless	¼ cup	130
Raspberries	fresh	1 cup	64
Rice, brown	cooked	1 cup	216

Food	Type	Serving	Calories
Rice, white	cooked	1 cup	242
Roast beef	deli meat	1 oz.	30
Romaine lettuce	fresh	1 cup, chopped	10
Salmon, wild	cooked	3 oz.	156
Salsa		1 tbsp.	4
Saltine cracker		1 cracker	13
Sausage, Italian	cooked	3 oz.	125
Sausage, pork	cooked	1 link, 4" long	44
Scallops, sea	cooked	6 large	120
Shrimp	cooked	4 large	22
Soda, Pepsi	regular	8 oz.	100
Soup	cream-based	1 cup	213
Soup	broth-based	1 cup	100
Sour cream	reduced-fat	1 tbsp.	20
Soybeans	boiled	1 cup	264
Soy milk	plain	1 cup	132
Spaghetti	cooked	1 cup	221
Spaghetti sauce	Alfredo	1 cup	480
Spaghetti sauce	marinara	1 cup	218
Spaghetti sauce	pesto	1 cup	920
Spinach	cooked	½ cup	20
Spinach	raw	1 cup	10
Squash, butternut	cooked	1 cup	80
Squash, spaghetti	cooked	1 cup	40
Steak, filet mignon	broiled	4 oz.	202
Steak, sirloin	broiled	4 oz.	212
Strawberries	fresh	1 cup, halves	48
String cheese	light, packaged	1 piece	60
Sugar	granulated	1 tsp.	16
Sugar	granulated	1 packet	11
Sweet potato	baked	1 medium	103
Sweet potato fries	baked	1 medium	103
Syrup	maple	1 tbsp.	52
Tartar sauce	regular	1 tbsp.	40
Tea, green	brewed	1 tea bag	0
Tilapia	cooked	3 oz.	110
Tofu	firm, raw	¼ block	117
Tomato	raw	1 medium	15
Tomato juice	with salt added	1 cup	41

Food	Type	Serving	Calories
Top sirloin	lean, cooked	3 oz.	158
Tortilla, corn	soft taco	1 6-inch	45
Tortilla, flour	soft taco	1 6-inch	110
Tortilla, flour	soft taco	1 8-inch	146
Tortilla, flour	burrito	1 10-inch	210
Tortilla chips	corn	1 oz.	140
Tuna	in oil	5 oz. can	220
Tuna	in water, no salt	5 oz. can	100
Tuna, yellowfin	fresh	3 oz.	121
Turkey breast	deli meat	1 oz.	28
Turkey, dark meat	no skin, cooked	3 oz.	160
Turkey, ground	99% fat-free	4 oz.	120
Turkey, light meat	no skin, cooked	3 oz.	120
Vegetable juice	low sodium	1 cup	50
Waffle	Eggo Nutri-Grain	1 4″ round	71
Walnuts	roasted	1 oz.	185
Water	regular	8 oz.	0
Whey protein	powder	1 scoop	120
Wine	red	4 oz.	108
Wine	white	4 oz.	89
Yam	baked	½ cup	79
Yogurt, plain	fat-free	6 oz.	75
Yogurt	fruit on bottom	6 oz.	150
Yogurt, frozen	fat-free	½ cup	110
Yogurt, Greek	fat-free	6 oz.	90
Zucchini	cooked	1 cup	30

APPENDIX D
BRAIN HEALTHY SHOPPING GUIDE

If you're worried that trying to follow a brain healthy nutrition plan will restrict you to only a few foods, then I have good news for you! There are literally thousands of brain healthy foods that taste great.

To make it easier for you to start or stay on track with your brain healthy eating program, I have created a shopping list with nearly two hundred of my favorite brain healthy foods. The items on this list are included because they meet one or more of the following brain healthy criteria.

- Lean protein
- Low glycemic
- High in fiber
- Low sodium
- Healthy fats
- High-quality calories
- Brain healthy spices
- Healthy liquids

Make a copy of this list and check off your favorites before you go to the grocery store so you can stock up on delicious brain healthy foods. Whenever possible, I would highly recommend that you choose foods that are organic, hormone-free, and antibiotic-free.

Foods with an asterisk are one of the Fifty Best Brain Healthy Foods.

BRAIN HEALTHY SHOPPING LIST

PRODUCE

- ☐ Acorn squash
- ☐ Apples*
- ☐ Apricots
- ☐ Artichokes
- ☐ Asparagus*
- ☐ Avocados*
- ☐ Bananas*
- ☐ Bell peppers
  (yellow, green, red,
  orange)*
- ☐ Beets*
- ☐ Blackberries*
- ☐ Blueberries*
- ☐ Bok choy*
- ☐ Broccoli*
- ☐ Brussels sprouts*
- ☐ Butternut squash
- ☐ Cabbage
- ☐ Cantaloupe
- ☐ Carrots
- ☐ Cauliflower
- ☐ Celery
- ☐ Cherries*
- ☐ Coconut*

- ☐ Collard greens
- ☐ Corn
- ☐ Cranberries
- ☐ Cucumbers
- ☐ Eggplant
- ☐ Goji berries*
- ☐ Grapefruit*
- ☐ Green beans
- ☐ Honeydew
- ☐ Jicama
- ☐ Kale
- ☐ Kiwi*
- ☐ Leeks
- ☐ Lemons*
- ☐ Lettuce
- ☐ Limes*
- ☐ Mangoes
- ☐ Mesclun
- ☐ Mushrooms
- ☐ Mustard greens
- ☐ Nectarines
- ☐ Okra
- ☐ Onions
- ☐ Oranges*

- ☐ Papaya
- ☐ Parsnips
- ☐ Peaches*
- ☐ Pears*
- ☐ Peas*
- ☐ Plums*
- ☐ Pomegranates*
- ☐ Pumpkin
- ☐ Radish
- ☐ Raspberries*
- ☐ Red grapes*
- ☐ Snap peas
- ☐ Soybeans*
- ☐ Spaghetti squash
- ☐ Spinach*
- ☐ Strawberries*
- ☐ Swiss chard
- ☐ Tangerines
- ☐ Tomatoes*
- ☐ Turnips
- ☐ Watercress
- ☐ Yams/sweet
  potatoes*
- ☐ Zucchini

MEATS & SEAFOOD

- ☐ Anchovies
- ☐ Beef, lean cuts
- ☐ Chicken, ground
  white meat
- ☐ Chicken, skinless*
- ☐ Clams
- ☐ Crab
- ☐ Flounder
- ☐ Haddock

- ☐ Halibut
- ☐ Herring*
- ☐ Lamb
- ☐ Lobster
- ☐ Mackerel
- ☐ Oysters
- ☐ Salmon, wild*
- ☐ Sardines
- ☐ Scallops

- ☐ Sea bass
- ☐ Shrimp
- ☐ Snapper
- ☐ Swordfish
- ☐ Trout
- ☐ Tuna*
- ☐ Turkey, ground
  white meat
- ☐ Turkey, skinless*

REFRIGERATED PRODUCTS

- ☐ Cheese, low/nonfat
- ☐ Cottage cheese, low/nonfat
- ☐ Egg whites, DHA-enriched*
- ☐ Egg substitutes
- ☐ Guacamole
- ☐ Hummus
- ☐ Salsa
- ☐ Tofu
- ☐ Yogurt, unsweetened*

BEVERAGES

- ☐ Almond milk, unsweetened*
- ☐ Coffee (decaf)
- ☐ Rice milk, unsweetened
- ☐ Soy milk, unsweetened
- ☐ Tea, black (decaf)
- ☐ Tea, green* (decaf)
- ☐ Tea, herbal (decaf)
- ☐ Water*

BEANS

- ☐ Black beans*
- ☐ Black-eyed peas
- ☐ Fava beans
- ☐ Kidney beans
- ☐ Pinto beans*
- ☐ Garbanzo beans*
- ☐ Lentils*
- ☐ Lima beans
- ☐ Navy beans
- ☐ Soybeans (edamame)
- ☐ Split peas
- ☐ White beans

BREADS, CEREALS, AND GRAINS

- ☐ Barley*
- ☐ Brown rice
- ☐ Bulgur (cracked wheat)
- ☐ Oats*
- ☐ Quinoa*
- ☐ Whole wheat bread
- ☐ Whole wheat flour
- ☐ Whole wheat tortillas

NUTS AND OILS

- ☐ Almond butter
- ☐ Almonds
- ☐ Almonds, raw*
- ☐ Coconut oil*
- ☐ Cashews
- ☐ Flaxseed oil
- ☐ Hazelnuts
- ☐ Olive oil*
- ☐ Olive oil spray
- ☐ Pecans
- ☐ Pistachios
- ☐ Pumpkin seeds
- ☐ Sesame seeds
- ☐ Sunflower seeds
- ☐ Walnuts*

SPICES, SEASONINGS, AND DRESSINGS

- ☐ Balsamic vinegar
- ☐ Balsamic vinaigrette, low-fat/low-sugar
- ☐ Basil
- ☐ Cinnamon
- ☐ Curry/turmeric
- ☐ Garlic
- ☐ Ginger
- ☐ Marinara sauce, low-fat/low-sugar
- ☐ Marjoram
- ☐ Mustard
- ☐ Oregano
- ☐ Rosemary
- ☐ Saffron
- ☐ Sage
- ☐ Thyme

SNACKS AND HEALTH FOODS

- ☐ Applesauce, unsweetened
- ☐ Dark chocolate, low sugar

- ☐ Dried veggies, no added oil
- ☐ Stevia
- ☐ Whey protein

- ☐ Xylitol

FROZEN FOODS

- ☐ Chicken breasts
- ☐ Fruits

- ☐ Seafood
- ☐ Turkey burgers

- ☐ Veggie burgers
- ☐ Veggies

APPENDIX E
BRAIN HEALTHY RECIPES

Eating brain healthy meals doesn't mean you have to give up flavor. Eating in a brain healthy way is about abundance, not deprivation. It is about great taste and wise spending. Your attitude here is critical. If you think of it as a loss of lasagna, you will not stick with it. But when you think of eating right as a *gain* in energy, a *gain* in happiness, a *gain* in brainpower, and a *gain* in time with your loved ones, you are much more likely to stay on track.

The recipes here can help you get thinner, smarter, and happier. In each recipe, I have highlighted the ingredients that can be found on the lists of the Fifty Best Brain Healthy Foods, Good Mood Foods (foods that make you thinner and happier), and Get Smart Foods (foods that make you thinner and smarter) to help you find the best recipes for your needs. Plus, I have highlighted the brain healthy—and virtually no-calorie—spices that will boost your brain and your mood.

All of these brain healthy recipes have been taste-tested by yours truly, and I can tell you they are delicious. Some of them come from the *Change Your Brain, Change Your Body Cookbook,* written by my beautiful wife, Tana, who has worked as a neurosurgical ICU nurse and who has been focused on health, fitness, and nutrition for over two decades. Some of them are from Tana's newest book, *The Amen Solution Cookbook,* which will help you incorporate the principles in this book so you can eat right to think right to get thinner, smarter, and happier. The following recipes are just a taste of what you will find in these wonderful brain healthy cookbooks.

I hope this will whet your appetite to get creative and started coming up with your own brain healthy recipes. If you do, please share them with us on our website.

BREAKFAST

DANIEL'S BREAKFAST SHAKE
(from *Change Your Brain, Change Your Body Cookbook*)

INGREDIENTS

Dr. Amen's Brain Boost Mix (20 grams of rice protein, plus a wonderful mix of a multiple vitamin and brain nutrients)

20 ounces water

1 cup frozen organic blueberries

1 cup frozen mixed fruit

Cinnamon-flavored liquid stevia to taste (using too much stevia can produce a bitter taste, so start with just a few drops)

1 scoop Green Vibrance (freeze-dried greens)

PREPARATION

1. Place all ingredients in a blender and mix well.
2. Serve chilled.

Serves 2
Calories per serving: 136.5

BRAIN BOOSTERS

Fifty Best Brain Foods: water, blueberries, fruit
Good Mood Foods: protein
Get Smart Foods: blueberries, water, fruit, cinnamon
Brain healthy spices: cinnamon

ALMOND BUTTER QUINOA
(from *Change Your Brain, Change Your Body Cookbook*)

INGREDIENTS

1 cup quinoa, rinsed

2 cups unsweetened almond milk or rice milk

2 tablespoons chunky almond butter

¼ teaspoon cinnamon

¼ teaspoon maple extract

¼ cup raisins (optional)

1 banana, thinly sliced

2 tablespoons slivered almonds

1 packet dry stevia (optional)

½ cup any other brain healthy fresh fruit topping of your choice

PREPARATION

1. In a medium saucepan over high heat, bring the quinoa, milk, almond butter, cinnamon, and maple extract to a boil.

2. Reduce heat, cover, and simmer until milk is absorbed, about 15 minutes.

3. Turn off heat and add the raisins. Let stand for 5 minutes.

4. Add the banana, almonds, and stevia, if desired.

5. Top with fresh fruit and serve warm.

Serves 4

Calories per serving: 205

BRAIN BOOSTERS

Fifty Best Brain Foods: quinoa, unsweetened almond milk, bananas, almonds, fruit
Good Mood Foods: almonds and almond butter (nuts), bananas
Get Smart Foods: cinnamon
Brain healthy spices: cinnamon

DR. AMEN'S LOW-FAT SOUTHWESTERN CHICKEN OMELET

INGREDIENTS

1 tablespoon extra-virgin olive oil

3 ounces lean turkey or chicken, chopped

6 egg whites or Egg Beaters

½ chopped tomato

1 handful mushrooms

Chopped onions, to taste

1 cup chopped red bell pepper

1 ounce low-fat mozzarella cheese, shredded

PREPARATION

1. If the chicken or turkey is not precooked, cook it first in a separate pan.

2. Preheat the oven on broil to 450 degrees F.

3. Add oil to skillet, pour in egg whites or Egg Beaters, and cook over medium heat for a minute or so.

4. Mix the vegetables together with the meat and add to the egg skillet. Cook until the eggs are as you like them.

5. Remove from heat.

6. Sprinkle the cheese on top of the omelet.

7. Put the skillet in the oven and bake for several minutes until the cheese is lightly browned.

Serves 2
Calories per serving: 200

BRAIN BOOSTERS

Fifty Best Brain Foods: egg whites, tomatoes, red bell peppers, lean turkey or chicken, olive oil
Good Mood Foods: eggs, protein, cheese
Get Smart Foods: eggs, tomatoes, red bell peppers, turkey, chicken

---

FEEL-GOOD EGGS RANCHERO
(from *The Amen Solution Cookbook*)

INGREDIENTS

1 tablespoon coconut oil

2 shallots, chopped

1 garlic clove, minced

½ cup canned black beans, drained and rinsed

½ teaspoon cumin

½ teaspoon paprika

1 egg plus 2 egg whites, or substitute Egg Beaters for the eggs, using the equivalent of 3 to 4 eggs

Real Salt and freshly ground black pepper (I love the Real Salt brand of salt, which has no additives or chemicals and has not been heat processed)

2 whole wheat or sprouted grain tortillas (you may prefer gluten-free tortillas, which can be found at most health food stores)

4 tablespoons fire-roasted salsa

PREPARATION

1. In a medium nonstick skillet, heat the oil over medium heat. Sauté the shallots and garlic for three minutes.

2. Add the beans, cumin, and paprika and cook for 4 minutes, stirring frequently.

3. In a small bowl, whisk the egg and egg whites and add to the beans.

4. Season with salt and pepper. Cook for about 2 minutes, until eggs begin to firm up.

5. Warm the tortillas in the microwave for 30 seconds or heat in a separate pan, turning frequently.

6. Transfer to a plate, top with the egg and bean mixture, and serve with salsa.

Serves 2
Calories per serving: 200

BRAIN BOOSTERS

Fifty Best Brain Foods: egg whites, black beans, tomatoes (in the salsa), coconut oil
Good Mood Foods: beans, eggs
Get Smart Foods: eggs, whole grains, tomatoes (in the salsa)
Brain healthy spices: garlic

RED, WHITE, AND BLUE SMOOTHIE

INGREDIENTS

½ cup plain nonfat, unsweetened yogurt
2 tablespoons flaxseed oil
Stevia, to taste
½ Gala or Washington apple
¼ cup frozen strawberries
1 cup frozen blueberries

PREPARATION

1. Place all ingredients in blender and mix well.
2. Serve chilled.

Serves 2
Calories per serving: 250

BRAIN BOOSTERS

Fifty Best Brain Foods: yogurt, apples, strawberries, blueberries
Good Mood Foods: protein (in the yogurt)
Get Smart Foods: apples, strawberries, blueberries

BRAIN BERRY DECADENCE

INGREDIENTS

8 ounces frozen mixed berries (blueberries, raspberries, and blackberries)
6 ounces nonfat sugar-free plain yogurt
¼ cup All-Bran cereal
1 tablespoon chopped walnuts (for crunch and omega-3 fatty acids)
1 tablespoon whey protein

PREPARATION

1. Heat the frozen berries in the microwave, then stir in the yogurt, cereal, walnuts, and protein.

2. Eat warm. It tastes like pie filling but is very healthy, with three of our favorite foods.

Serves 1
Calories per serving: 230

BRAIN BOOSTERS

Fifty Best Brain Foods: blueberries, raspberries, blackberries, yogurt, walnuts
Good Mood Foods: protein (in the yogurt), nuts
Get Smart Foods: blueberries, raspberries, blackberries, walnuts, whole grains (All-Bran cereal)

LUNCH

SMART SPINACH SALAD

INGREDIENTS

2 cups fresh spinach
1 handful walnuts
3 strawberries, sliced
1 hard-boiled egg white, sliced

3 ounces turkey breast, cooked and chopped
½ avocado, sliced
2 tablespoons Newman's Own Lighten Up Balsamic Vinaigrette Dressing

PREPARATION

1. Mix the ingredients together and serve.

Serves 1
Calories per serving: 425

BRAIN BOOSTERS

50 Best Brain Foods: spinach, walnuts, strawberries, egg whites, turkey, avocado
Good Mood Foods: spinach, walnuts, eggs, protein
Get Smart Foods: spinach, walnuts, strawberries, eggs, avocados, turkey

---

MAGNIFICENT MIND CUCUMBER MINT SALAD
(from *Change Your Brain, Change Your Body Cookbook*)

INGREDIENTS

1 bunch mint, stems removed
1 bunch parsley, stems removed
2 cucumbers, minced
1 red bell pepper, finely chopped
6 scallions (white and green parts), minced
4 tomatoes, seeded and finely chopped
½ cup fresh lemon juice
¼ cup olive oil
½ teaspoon Real Salt
½ teaspoon paprika

PREPARATION

1. Mince the mint and parsley finely by hand or in food processor if preferred.

2. In large mixing bowl, combine the herbs with the cucumbers, bell pepper, scallions, and tomatoes.

3. Add the lemon juice, olive oil, Real Salt, and paprika.

4. Toss and serve.

Serves 6
Calories per serving: 130

BRAIN BOOSTERS

Fifty Best Brain Foods: red bell pepper, tomatoes, lemons, olive oil
Good Mood Foods: lemons
Get Smart Foods: red bell peppers, tomatoes

MINDFUL MINESTRONE SOUP
(from *The Amen Solution Cookbook*)

INGREDIENTS

2 tablespoons olive oil
1 onion, coarsely chopped
2 celery stalks, chopped
2 small potatoes, cubed
1 carrot, chopped
1 zucchini, sliced
1 teaspoon fresh thyme, chopped
1 bay leaf
1 15-ounce can organic stewed tomatoes
4 cups vegetable stock
1 15-ounce can organic kidney beans, drained and rinsed
½ cup dry pasta, whole wheat or gluten-free
2 cups fresh baby spinach
2 tablespoons finely chopped fresh parsley
Real Salt and freshly ground black pepper

PREPARATION

1. In a large pot, heat the olive oil over medium heat.
2. Stir in the onion, celery, potatoes, and carrot. Cook, stirring frequently, for about 5 minutes.
3. Stir in the zucchini, thyme, and bay leaf and cook for another 2 minutes.
4. Add the tomatoes and stock. Bring to a boil, reduce heat, and simmer for 10 minutes.
5. Stir in the beans and pasta and simmer for 10 minutes.
6. Add spinach and parsley. Season with salt and pepper.
7. Serve hot.

Serves 4
Calories per serving: 250

BRAIN BOOSTERS

Fifty Best Brain Foods: olive oil, carrots, tomatoes, beans, spinach
Good Mood Foods: beans, spinach
Get Smart Foods: beans, spinach, thyme, tomatoes, whole grains
Brain healthy spices: thyme

BRAIN FITNESS FAJITA SALAD
(from *The Amen Solution Cookbook*)

INGREDIENTS

2 tablespoons olive oil

1 lime, juiced

2 garlic cloves, minced

1 teaspoon ground cumin

1 teaspoon chopped fresh oregano

2 boneless, skinless chicken breasts (6–8 ounces), cut into thin strips

1 onion, cut into wedges

1 red bell pepper, cut into thin strips

1 can organic chopped green chili peppers

Romaine lettuce, leaves separated

3 tomatoes, cut into wedges

1 avocado, sliced

2 tablespoons cilantro, chopped

1 15-ounce can organic black or pinto beans, drained and rinsed
     (optional)

2 tablespoons organic salsa (optional)

Baked organic tortilla chips

Sunflower seeds (optional)

Dairy-free or nonfat sour cream (optional)

PREPARATION

1. In a large bowl, combine 1 tablespoon of the olive oil, the lime juice, garlic, cumin, and oregano.

2. Add the chicken to the bowl and marinate for 1 to 24 hours.

3. Heat the remaining tablespoon of olive oil in a nonstick skillet over medium to medium-high heat.

4. Add the onion and sauté for 2 minutes.

5. Remove the chicken from marinade and add to skillet. Cook for 7 minutes, turning every couple of minutes.

6. Add the red bell pepper and chili peppers. Cook for an additional 3 minutes, or until the chicken is cooked through.

7. Serve over lettuce leaves and top with the tomatoes, avocado, and cilantro.

8. Add the beans, if desired, and top with salsa.

9. Crunch up a few tortilla chips and sprinkle over the top.

10. Add a few sunflower seeds and a dollop of sour cream, if desired.

Vegetarians can prepare this salad without the chicken. There is enough protein with the beans.

Serves 4
Calories per serving: 300

BRAIN BOOSTERS

Fifty Best Brain Foods: skinless chicken, olive oil, limes, bell peppers, tomatoes, avocado, black or pinto beans

Good Mood Foods: beans, chicken, sunflower seeds

Get Smart Foods: avocado, beans, skinless chicken, red bell peppers, tomatoes

Brain healthy spices: garlic, oregano

VERY VEGGIE SANDWICH

INGREDIENTS

2 slices whole wheat bread
1 slice low-fat Jack cheese, cut in 4 pieces
3–4 spinach leaves
½ tomato, sliced
1 mild green chili, sliced
½ red bell pepper, julienned
¼ cucumber, sliced, for garnish

PREPARATION

1. Put the veggies and cheese on bread slices.
2. Grill in George Foreman grill for 4 to 5 minutes.
3. Serve with cucumber garnish.

Serves 1
Calories per serving: 350

DINNER

TANA'S SMOOTH SWEET POTATO SOUP
(from *Change Your Brain, Change Your Body Cookbook*)

INGREDIENTS

6–7 cups vegetable stock

½ cup diced onion

⅓ cup diced celery

3 tablespoons diced leeks

2 garlic cloves, minced

1½ pounds sweet potatoes, peeled and diced

1 cinnamon stick

¼ teaspoon nutmeg

½ cup unsweetened almond milk

1 teaspoon Real Salt

1 teaspoon white pepper

2 tablespoons finely chopped fresh sage

⅛ cup cranberries

Cinnamon, sprinkled for garnish

¼ cup sunflower seeds (optional)

PREPARATION

1. Heat ¼ cup of the stock in large soup pot over medium heat. Sauté the onion, celery, and leeks for 2 minutes. Add the garlic and sauté for about 1 minute.

2. Add 4 cups of stock, sweet potatoes, cinnamon stick, and nutmeg. Bring to a boil then reduce heat to medium-low and simmer until the potatoes are tender, about 10 minutes.

3. Remove the cinnamon stick.

4. Use an immersion blender and blend until smooth (or pour contents into a blender in batches).

5. Pour the soup back into pot (if using a blender). Add the almond milk. Then slowly add the remaining stock according to preferred consistency.

6. Add the Real Salt and pepper.

7. Dish soup into bowls. Sprinkle with the sage, cranberries, and cinnamon and top with sunflower seeds, if desired.

8. Serve hot.

A BEAUTIFUL MARRIAGE

This soup tastes better when spices and herbs have a chance to marry with the vegetables. If time allows, remove from heat and allow soup to sit for 30 to 60 minutes. Then gently heat over low heat prior to serving.

Serves 8
Calories per serving: 81

BRAIN BOOSTERS

Fifty Best Brain Healthy Foods: sweet potatoes, unsweetened almond milk
Good Mood Foods: sunflower seeds
Get Smart Foods: cinnamon, sage, cranberries
Brain healthy spices: garlic, cinnamon, sage

GET SMART MAHI MAHI BURGER WITH PINEAPPLE SALSA
(from *The Amen Solution Cookbook*)

INGREDIENTS
1 cup diced fresh pineapple
½ cup diced red bell pepper
2 tablespoons minced fresh cilantro
1 tablespoon minced shallot
Real Salt and freshly ground black pepper
4 mahi mahi fillets (4 ounces each)
1 tablespoon coconut oil, melted
1 teaspoon white pepper
4 whole wheat or whole grain buns (I prefer the thin buns that are only 100 calories for the entire bun)

PREPARATION FOR SALSA

1. Mix the pineapple, bell pepper, cilantro, and shallot. Season with salt and black pepper.

2. Set aside.

PREPARATION FOR MAHI MAHI

1. Preheat the grill to medium hot.

2. Brush the fillets with the melted coconut oil and sprinkle with white pepper.

3. Grill the fillets for about 5 minutes per side or until mahi mahi flakes easily when tested with fork.

4. Serve on whole wheat bun with the pineapple salsa.

Serves 4
Calories per serving: 350

BRAIN BOOSTERS

Fifty Best Brain Healthy Foods: red bell peppers, coconut oil
Good Mood Foods: seafood
Get Smart Foods: red bell peppers, whole grains

JT'S GRILLED SALMON

INGREDIENTS

4 lemon slices
½ each red and yellow bell pepper
Onions, sliced, to taste
1 salmon fillet (about 3 ounces)
Lemon pepper, to taste
Real Salt, to taste

PREPARATION

1. Arrange the lemon slices, bell peppers, and onion on a piece of foil and lay the fish on top.

2. Wrap loosely, and make a short tent to seal it.

3. Place on grill at medium heat or in oven at 375 degrees F and cook until done, about 20 minutes.

4. Sprinkle with Real Salt and lemon pepper and serve.

Serves 1
Calories per serving: 200

HEALTHY TURKEY CHILI
(from *Change Your Brain, Change Your Body Cookbook*)

INGREDIENTS
1 tablespoon refined coconut oil
1 pound lean ground turkey (free-range, hormone-free)
1 cup chopped onion
3 garlic cloves, chopped
1 jalapeño pepper (optional)
1 teaspoon chili powder
1 4-ounce can Ortega chilis
1 tablespoon chopped fresh oregano
1 teaspoon cumin seed
1–2 teaspoons Real Salt
3 cups diced tomatoes, fresh or organic canned (no-salt-added variety)
2 cups chicken or vegetable stock
1 cup chopped bell pepper
½ cup chopped zucchini
2 cups chopped celery
2 cups cooked kidney beans
1 cup cooked black beans or chickpeas

PREPARATION
1. In a large saucepan or pot, brown the turkey meat in the coconut oil over medium heat. Crumble the turkey, breaking it apart as much as possible. Add the onion, stirring for about 2 minutes.

2. Add the garlic, jalapeño (if using), chili powder, chilis, oregano, cumin seed, Real Salt, and tomatoes. Mix thoroughly until spices are well blended with the meat.

3. Add the stock.

4. Dish out 2 cups of the chili mixture. Put 1 cup of chili at a time into the blender. Add ½ cup of chopped bell pepper, zucchini, and celery at a time and purée. Pour mixture back into the remaining chili pot. (Adding

the puréed vegetables not only makes the chili tasty but is a great way to add fiber and vitamins without overcooking.)

5. Add the kidney beans and black beans. Stir thoroughly and heat through on medium-low, about 5 minutes.

6. Serve hot.

Serves 8

Calories per serving: 209

BRAIN BOOSTERS

Fifty Best Brain Foods: turkey, tomatoes, bell peppers, beans, coconut oil

Good Mood Foods: protein (turkey), beans

Get Smart Foods: turkey, tomatoes, red bell peppers, beans

Brain healthy spices: garlic

SAVORY LUBIAN ROSE LAMB STEW
(from *The Amen Solution Cookbook*)

INGREDIENTS

½ cup barley

¼ teaspoon Real Salt

¼ teaspoon pepper

½ teaspoon cinnamon

1 tablespoon refined coconut oil

½ small onion, chopped

12 ounces lean lamb (grass-fed, antibiotic-free, hormone-free), chopped into bite-size pieces

28-ounce can diced tomatoes

¼ teaspoon pepper

2 cups fresh green beans, trimmed

2 tablespoons toasted pine nuts (optional)

PREPARATION

1. Place barley in 1 cup of boiling water. Add the salt, pepper, and cinnamon. Cook according to time on package, approximately 30 to 45 minutes.

2. Heat the coconut oil in medium-large pan over medium heat. Add the onion and sauté for one minute.

3. Add the lamb and cook until meat is lightly browned, about 5 minutes.

4. Add the tomatoes and pepper. Simmer for 15 minutes.

5. Add the green beans and simmer for 5 minutes.

6. Place the cooked barley on serving platter and serve lamb mixture over the top.

7. Sprinkle with pine nuts, if desired.

Serves 4
Calories per serving: 350

BRAIN BOOSTERS

Fifty Best Brain Foods: tomatoes, barley, coconut oil
Good Mood Foods: lamb (lean meats/protein), nuts
Get Smart Foods: barley, pine nuts, tomatoes
Brain healthy spices: cinnamon

DESSERT

EZ BLUEBERRY ICE CREAM
(from *Change Your Brain, Change Your Body Cookbook*)

INGREDIENTS

16 ounces frozen blueberries

8 ounces coconut yogurt

10 drops plain or vanilla-flavored stevia

PREPARATION

1. Mix all the ingredients in a large bowl.

2. Dish into dessert bowls and serve cold.

Serves 2
Calories per serving: 97

BRAIN BOOSTERS

Fifty Best Brain Foods: blueberries, yogurt
Good Mood Foods: protein (in the yogurt)
Get Smart Foods: blueberries

SCINTILLATING SUGAR-FREE SORBET
(from *Change Your Brain, Change Your Body Cookbook*)

INGREDIENTS

Zest and juice of 1 lemon
½ cup sliced fresh strawberries
½ cup fresh raspberries
1 cup fresh blueberries
5–10 drops vanilla-flavored stevia, to taste
Shaved coconut, for topping (optional)

PREPARATION

1. Add the lemon zest and juice, and strawberries, raspberries, and blueberries to a blender. Blend for 30 to 60 seconds.

2. Add the stevia a couple drops at a time.

3. Blend until smooth.

4. Serve immediately.

FOR ICE CREAM MAKER

1. Add the lemon zest and juice, and strawberries, raspberries, and blueberries to a blender and purée.

2. Pour the fruit mixture through metal strainer. Discard the pulp and seeds.

3. Add the stevia a couple drops at a time and mix.

4. Follow instructions on ice cream maker to freeze fruit mixture. This usually takes several hours.

Serves 2
Calories per serving: 80

BRAIN BOOSTERS

Fifty Best Brain Healthy Foods: lemons, strawberries, raspberries, blueberries, coconut
Good Mood Foods: lemons
Get Smart Foods: strawberries, raspberries, blueberries

APPENDIX F

CALORIES BURNED FROM PHYSICAL ACTIVITY

Activity (1-hour duration)	100 lbs.	130 lbs.	160 lbs.	200 lbs.	240 lbs.	270 lbs.	300 lbs.
Aerobics, high impact	318	413	511	637	763	859	954
Aerobics, low impact	276	359	365	455	545	745	828
Basketball, full court	498	647	584	728	872	1,345	1,494
Bowling	138	179	219	273	327	373	414
Burst training	266	342	424	532	642	720	794
Dancing	138	179	219	273	327	373	414
Elliptical trainer	516	671	826	1,032	1,238	1,393	1,548
Golf, carry clubs	276	359	329	410	491	745	828
Hiking	270	351	438	546	654	729	810
Jogging 5 mph	384	499	614	768	922	1,037	1,152
Jogging 6 mph	456	593	730	912	1,094	1,231	1,368
Jogging 7 mph	522	679	835	1,044	1,253	1,409	1,566
Rope jumping	456	593	730	910	1,090	1,231	1,368
Rowing machine	318	413	511	637	763	859	954
Ski machine	439	569	701	876	1,051	1,183	1,314

Activity (1-hour duration)	100 lbs.	130 lbs.	160 lbs.	200 lbs.	240 lbs.	270 lbs.	300 lbs.
Soccer (no heading!)	318	413	509	636	763	859	954
Softball or baseball	228	296	365	455	545	616	684
Stair step machine	318	413	513	636	763	859	954
Stationary bike	318	413	509	636	763	859	954
Step aerobics	480	624	768	960	1,152	1,296	1,440
Swimming	276	359	511	637	763	745	828
Table tennis	180	234	288	360	432	486	540
Tae kwon do	456	593	730	910	1,090	1,231	1,368
Tai chi	108	144	292	364	436	490	544
Tennis, doubles	192	250	307	384	461	518	576
Tennis, singles	276	359	584	728	872	745	828
Volleyball	156	203	292	364	436	421	468
Walking 2 mph	126	164	183	228	273	340	378
Walking 3 mph	198	257	317	396	475	535	594
Walking 3.5 mph	181	235	277	346	414	584	649
Walking 4 mph	234	304	374	468	562	632	702
Weight lifting	156	203	219	273	327	421	468

APPENDIX G

EAT ECO-FRIENDLY
BRAIN HEALTHY FOODS

Not all foods are created equal, not even brain healthy foods. Part of brain healthy eating is being smart about choosing the foods that are the best not only for our brains and bodies but also for the environment. When shopping for the brain healthy fish included on the Brain Healthy Shopping List, choose the most eco-friendly. The following recommendations come from the Monterey Bay Aquarium Seafood Watch program. You can download pocket guides to more types of fish at: www.montereybayaquarium.org/cr/cr_seafoodwatch/download.aspx.

Brain Healthy Fish	Eat These Often	Okay to Eat Sometimes	Don't Eat These
Clams	farmed	wild	
Crab	Dungeness, Stone	Blue, King (U.S.), Snow	
Flounder		Pacific	Atlantic
Halibut	Pacific		Atlantic
Herring		Atlantic	
Lobster	Spiny (U.S.)	American/Maine	Spiny (Brazil)
Oysters	farmed	wild	

Brain Healthy Fish	Eat These Often	Okay to Eat Sometimes	Don't Eat These
Salmon	wild (Alaska)	wild (Washington)	wild (California, Oregon); farmed, including Atlantic
Scallops	farmed off bottom	sea	
Seabass			Chilean seabass
Shrimp	Pink (Oregon)	U.S. or Canada	imported
Snapper			Red
Swordfish		U.S.	imported
Trout	Rainbow (farmed)		
Tuna	Albacore, including canned white tuna (pole/troll, U.S. and British Columbia); Skipjack including canned light tuna (pole/troll)	Bigeye, Yellowfin (pole/troll); canned white/Albacore (pole/troll except U.S. and British Columbia)	Albacore, Bigeye, Yellowfin (longline); Bluefin, Tongol; canned (except pole/troll)

APPENDIX H

FLASH CARDS

Keep These with You at All Times

Staying on track with your brain healthy lifestyle when you're at home is one thing. But as someone who travels *a lot*, I can tell you that sticking with it can be more challenging when you are on the road. I carry reminder cards with me everywhere I go. It helps me remember what to do. On the following pages are cards you can photocopy, cut out, and put in your wallet to carry with you so you will always be reminded about brain health. I hope you find them helpful.

SUGGESTED SERVINGS SIZES / EQUIVALENTS

Proteins

3 oz. meat/poultry	= 1 deck of cards
3 oz. grilled fish	= 1 checkbook
1 cup cooked beans	= 1 baseball
2 tbsp. peanut butter	= 1 Ping-Pong ball

Grains

½ cup cooked pasta, rice, or oatmeal	= 1 tennis ball
1 cup dry cereal	= your fist
1 slice bread	= 1 CD case

Dairy and Cheese

1 cup yogurt	= 1 baseball
1 ½ oz. cheese	= 4 dice

Vegetables and Fruits

1 cup raw leafy greens	= 1 baseball
½ cup cooked veggies	= 2 golf balls
1 medium apple/orange	= 1 tennis ball
½ cup fresh fruit	= 2 golf balls
¼ cup dried fruit	=1 large egg in shell

Fats

1 tsp. butter	= 1 dice
2 tbsp. salad dressing	= 1 Ping-Pong ball
1 oz. nuts	= 1 handful

Liquid Measures

1 gal. = 4 qt. = 8 pt. = 16 cups = 128 fl. oz.
½ gal. = 2 qt. = 4 pt. = 8 cups = 64 fl. oz.
¼ gal. = 1 qt. = 2 pt. = 4 cups = 32 fl oz.
½ qt. = 1 pt. = 2 cups = 16 fl. oz.
¼ qt. = ½ pt. = 1 cup = 8 fl oz.

Dry Measures

1 cup = 16 tbsp. = 48 tsp. = 250 ml

¾ cup = 12 tbsp. = 36 tsp. = 175 ml

⅔ cup = 10⅔ tbsp. = 32 tsp. = 150 ml

½ cup = 8 tbsp. = 24 tsp. = 125 ml

⅓ cup = 5⅓ tbsp. = 16 tsp. = 75 ml

¼ cup = 4 tbsp. = 12 tsp. = 50 ml

1 tbsp. = 3 tsp. = 15 ml

Quick Equivalency Chart

3 tsp. = 1 tbsp.

2 tbsp. = ⅛ cup = 1 fl. oz.

4 tbsp. = ¼ cup = 2 fl. oz.

5 tbsp. + 1 tsp. = ⅓ cup

8 tbsp. = ½ cup

1 cup = ½ pt.

2 cups = 1 pt.

4 cups = 2 pts. = 1 qt.

4 qt. = 1 gal.

16 oz. = 1 lb.

dash or pinch = less than ⅛ tsp.

DR. AMEN'S TYPE 1
COMPULSIVE OVEREATERS

(use if you have combo Types 1,4 / Types 1,5 / Types 1,4,5)

DO: aerobic exercise, vary workouts, distract yourself when stuck on negative thoughts, have options, meditate

EAT: brain healthy complex carbs

TAKE: 5-HTP, inositol, saffron, L-tryptophan, St. John's wort (Serotonin Mood Support)

DON'T: automatically say no; eat high-protein diets; consume caffeine, stimulants, and diet pills

DR. AMEN'S TYPE 2
IMPULSIVE OVEREATERS

(use if you have combo Types 2,4 / Types 2,5 / Types 2,4,5)

DO: aerobic exercise every day, choose activities you love, yoga, set clear goals, get outside supervision, meditate

EAT: brain healthy lean protein at every meal

TAKE: multivitamin, omega-3, vitamin D, green tea, rhodiola (Focus & Energy Optimizer)

DON'T: automatically say yes; eat high-carb diets; consume alcohol, caffeine, and sugar; stress

DR. AMEN'S TYPE 3
IMPULSIVE-COMPULSIVE OVEREATERS

(use if you have combo Types 3,4 / Types 3,5 / Types 3,4,5)

DO: aerobic exercise every day, choose activities you love, vary workouts, set goals, have options, distract yourself when stuck on negative thoughts

EAT: balanced brain healthy diet

TAKE: multivitamin, omega-3, vitamin D, combine green tea & 5-HTP (Serotonin Mood Support/Focus & Energy Optimizer)

DON'T: automatically say no or yes

DR. AMEN'S TYPE 4
SAD OR EMOTIONAL OVEREATERS

(use Type 4 and Type 5 cards if you have combo Types 4,5)

DO: social physical activities, kill ANTs, write 5 things that make you grateful every day, volunteer, improve relationships

EAT: balanced brain healthy diet

TAKE: multivitamin, omega-3, vitamin D, SAMe (SAMe Mood & Movement Support)

DON'T: get stuck in negative thinking patterns

DR. AMEN'S TYPE 5 ANXIOUS OVEREATERS

(use Type 4 and Type 5 cards if you have combo Types 4,5)

DO: aerobic workouts, yoga, tai chi, meditate, deep breathing, kill ANTs, self-hypnosis, hand warming

EAT: balanced brain healthy diet

TAKE: multivitamin, omega-3, vitamin D, B_6, lemon balm, magnesium, GABA (GABA Calming Support)

DON'T: focus on the negative; consume caffeine, stimulants, alcohol, sugar, simple carbs; stress

DR. AMEN'S BRAIN HEALTHY REMINDERS

- Review One-Page Miracle
- Take brain healthy supplements
- Drink water requirement
- Use relaxation techniques
- Write 5 things I'm grateful for
- Write 1 thing that motivates me
- Kill ANTs
- Do daily meditation
- Eat right/ count calories
- Get 30 minutes exercise
- Get 7 hours sleep
- Learn something new every day

DR. AMEN'S 50 BEST BRAIN HEALTHY FOODS

Almonds, raw	Lemons
Almond milk, unsweetened	Lentils
Apples	Limes
Asparagus	Oats
Avocados	Olive oil
Bananas	Oranges
Barley	Peas
Beans	Peaches
Beets	Pears
Bell peppers (any color)	Peas
Blackberries	Plums
Blueberries	Pomegranates
Bok choy	Quinoa
Broccoli	Raspberries
Brussels sprouts	Red grapes
Cherries	Salmon, wild
Chicken, skinless	Soybeans
Coconut	Spinach
Coconut oil	Strawberries
Egg whites, DHA enriched	Tomatoes
Goji berries	Tuna
Grapefruit	Turkey, skinless
Green tea	Walnuts
Herring	Water
Kiwi	Yams/sweet potatoes
	Yogurt, low-fat, unsweetened

NOTE ON REFERENCES
AND FURTHER READING

The information in *The Amen Solution* is based on more than four hundred sources, including scientific studies, books, interviews with medical and nutrition experts, interviews with our weight-loss group participants, statistics from government agencies and health organizations, and other reliable sources. Printed out, the references take up dozens of pages. In an effort to save a few trees, I have decided to place them exclusively on our website. I invite you to view them at www.amenclinics.com.

ACKNOWLEDGMENTS

I am grateful to myriad people who have been instrumental in making *The Amen Solution* a reality, especially all of the patients and professionals who have taught me so much about how the brain relates to the health of our bodies and minds. I am especially grateful to my writing partner, Frances Sharpe, who was invaluable in the process of designing and completing this book. She remains committed to our mission and is a very thoughtful, hardworking, talented woman. Also, Dr. Kristen Willeumier, our Director of Research at the Amen Clinics, was a wonderful resource for research, collaboration, and encouragement.

Other staff at Amen Clinics, Inc., as always, provided tremendous help and support during this process, especially my personal assistant Catherine Hanlon, Krystle Johnson, Sheri Denham, Ronnette Leonard, Dr. Ed Carels, Jackie Frattali, Dr. Joseph Annibali, and Dr. Lilly Somner. I also wish to thank our weight-loss group leaders at the Amen Clinics; Dr. Jeff Fortuna from California State University Fullerton for his contribution on the brain healthy eating on a budget section; Andy Newberg and Mark Waldman for their insights on meditation and mindful eating; all our NFL players, but especially Big Ed White, Ray White and his wife, Nancy, Roy Williams, and Cam Cleeland for sharing their personal stories; all our All-Stars for sharing their stories; and all our weight-loss participants for their tips and inspiration.

I also wish to thank my amazing literary team at Crown Archetype, especially my kind and thoughtful editor, Julia Pastore, and my publisher, Tina Constable. I am forever grateful to my literary agent, Faith Hamlin, who besides being one of my best friends, is a thoughtful, protective, creative mentor, along with Stephanie Diaz, our foreign rights agent. If you are reading this outside of the United States,

Stephanie made that happen. In addition, I am grateful to all of my friends and colleagues at public television stations across the country. Public television is a treasure to our country and I am grateful to be able to partner with stations to bring our message of hope and healing to you. And to Tana—my wife, my joy, and my best friend—who patiently listened to me for hours on end and gave many thoughtful suggestions on the book. I love all of you.

INDEX

ABOUT THE AUTHOR

Daniel G. Amen, M.D., is a physician, child and adult psychiatrist, brain imaging specialist, and *New York Times* bestselling author. He is the writer, producer, and host of four highly successful public television programs, raising more than $30 million for public television. He is a Distinguished Fellow of the American Psychiatric Association and the CEO and medical director of Amen Clinics in Newport Beach and Fairfield, California; Bellevue, Washington; and Reston, Virginia.

Amen Clinics is the world leader in applying brain imaging science to everyday clinical practice and has the world's largest database of functional scans related to behavior, now totaling more than 60,000.

Dr. Amen is the author of forty professional scientific articles and twenty-five books, including the *New York Times* bestsellers *Change Your Brain, Change Your Body; Change Your Brain, Change Your Life;* and *Magnificent Mind at Any Age.* He is also the author of *Unchain Your Brain, Wired for Success, Healing ADD, Healing the Hardware of the Soul, Making a Good Brain Great, The Brain in Love,* and the coauthor of *Healing Anxiety and Depression* and *Preventing Alzheimer's.*

Dr. Amen spearheads the groundbreaking Amen Clinics retired NFL player brain imaging study and is intimately involved with The Daniel Challenge, a project of Pastor Rick Warren and Saddleback Church to create brain healthy churches.

Dr. Amen has appeared on the *Dr. Oz Show,* the *Today* show, *Good Morning America, The View, The Rachael Ray Show, Larry King Live, The Early Show,* CNN, HBO, Discovery Channel, and many other national television and radio programs. His national public television shows include *Change Your Brain, Change Your Life; Magnificent Mind at Any Age; The Brain in Love;* and *Change Your Brain, Change Your Body.*

A small sample of the organizations Dr. Amen has spoken for include the National Security Agency, the National Science Foundation, Harvard's Learning and the Brain Conference, the Million Dollar Roundtable, Independent Retired Football Players Summit, and the Supreme Courts of Delaware, Ohio, and Wyoming. Dr. Amen has been featured in *Newsweek, Parade* magazine, the *New York Times Magazine, Men's Health,* and *Cosmopolitan.*

Dr. Amen is married, the father of four children, grandfather to Elias, and is an avid table tennis player.

AMEN CLINICS, INC.

Amen Clinics, Inc. (ACI) was established in 1989 by Daniel G. Amen, M.D. It specializes in innovative diagnosis and treatment planning for a wide variety of behavioral, learning, emotional and cognitive, and weight problems for children, teenagers, and adults. ACI has an international reputation for evaluating brain-behavior problems, such as ADD, depression, anxiety, school failure, brain trauma, obsessive-compulsive disorders, aggressiveness, marital conflict, cognitive decline, brain toxicity from drugs or alcohol, and obesity. Brain SPECT imaging is performed in the Clinics. ACI has the world's largest database of brain scans for behavioral problems.

ACI welcomes referrals from physicians, psychologists, social workers, marriage and family therapists, drug and alcohol counselors, and individual clients.

Amen Clinics, Inc., Newport Beach
4019 Westerly Pl., Suite 100
Newport Beach, CA 92660
(888) 564-2700

Amen Clinics, Inc., Fairfield
350 Chadbourne Rd.
Fairfield, CA 94585
(888) 564-2700

Amen Clinics, Inc., Northwest
616 120th Ave. NE, Suite C100
Bellevue, WA 98005
(888) 564-2700

Amen Clinics, Inc., DC
1875 Campus Commons Dr.
Reston, VA 20191
(888) 564-2700

www.amenclinic.com

AMENCLINIC.COM

Amenclinic.com is an educational interactive brain website geared toward mental health and medical professionals, educators, students, and the general public. It contains a wealth of information to help you learn about our clinics and the brain. The site contains more than three hundred color brain SPECT images, thousands of scientific abstracts on brain SPECT imaging for psychiatry, body mass index and calorie calculators, and much, much more.

VIEW HUNDREDS OF ASTONISHING COLOR 3-D BRAIN SPECT IMAGES ON

ADD, including the six subtypes
Aggression
Anxiety disorders
Brain trauma
Dementia and cognitive decline
Depression
Drug abuse
Obsessive-compulsive disorder
PMS
Seizures
Stroke